OMAD

ONE MEAL A DAY

Easy Delicious Recipes for Intermittent Fasting To Burn Fat, Lose Weight and Improve Health

MONALISA BLAKE

TABLE OF CONTENT

TABLE OF CONTENT 2

INTRODUCTION 5

UNDERSTAND THAT IT MIGHT TAKE SOMETIME TO ADJUST 5

Safety Considerations and Precautions 6

How to Follow the OMAD Diet Safely 7

CHAPTER ONE: 9

Getting Started with the OMAD Diet 9

Calculating Your Caloric Needs 9

Choosing the Right Foods for Your OMAD Meals 10

Meal Planning and Preparation Tips 12

Grocery Shopping for the OMAD Diet 13

CHAPTER TWO: OMAD DIET RECIPES 17

BREAKFAST RECIPES 17

Apple Cinnamon Overnight Oats: 17

Vegetable Breakfast Skillet: 18

Banana Oat Pancakes: 19

Spinach and Mushroom Frittata: 20

Peanut Butter and Banana Smoothie: 21

Sweet Potato Hash with Eggs: 22

Scrambled Eggs with Spinach and Tomatoes: 23

Greek Yogurt with Honey and Mixed Berries: 24

Quinoa Breakfast Bowl with Almond Milk and Berries: 24

Avocado Toast with Poached Egg: 25

CHAPTER THREE: 27

LUNCH RECIPES 27

Grilled Chicken Salad: 27

Quinoa Stuffed Bell Peppers: 28

Salmon and Asparagus Foil Pack: 29

Baked Lemon Herb Chicken: 30

Beef Stir-Fry with Broccoli: 31

Shrimp and Zucchini Noodles: 32

Lentil Soup with Vegetables: 33

Turkey Lettuce Wraps with Avocado: 34

Cauliflower Fried Rice with Tofu: 35

Veggie Frittata with Spinach and Feta: 36

CHAPTER FOUR: 37

DINNER RECIPES 37

Grilled Salmon with Roasted Vegetables: 37

Cauliflower Fried Rice with Shrimp: 39

Baked Chicken Breast with Quinoa Salad: 40

Turkey Meatballs with Zucchini Noodles: 41

Stir-Fried Tofu with Broccoli and Cashews: 43

Eggplant Parmesan with Mixed Greens Salad: 44

Lentil and Vegetable Soup: 46

Beef and Vegetable Stir-Fry: 47

Spaghetti Squash with Turkey Bolognese: 48

Grilled Portobello Mushrooms with Balsamic Glaze: 49

CHAPTER FIVE: **51**

OMAD Diet Snacks and Desserts **51**

Healthy Snacks Option **51**

Almonds: 51

Baby Carrots with Hummus: 51

Greek Yogurt with Honey: 52

Sliced Cucumbers with Cottage Cheese: 53

Apple Slices with Almond Butter: 54

Celery Sticks with Peanut Butter: 54

Hard-Boiled Eggs: 55

Cherry Tomatoes with Mozzarella Cheese: 55

Edamame Beans: 56

Whole Grain Crackers with Avocado: 56

Guilt-Free Desserts **57**

Fresh Fruit Salad: 57

Greek Yogurt Parfait with Granola and Berries: 58

Chia Seed Pudding with Coconut Milk and Mango: 58

Baked Apples with Cinnamon and a Dollop of Greek Yogurt: 60

Frozen Banana Slices Dipped in Dark Chocolate: 61

Mixed Berry Sorbet Made with Frozen Berries and a Splash of Lemon Juice: 62

Coconut Milk Panna Cotta with Raspberry Coulis: 63

Chocolate Avocado Mousse: 64

Baked Peaches with a Sprinkle of Cinnamon and a Drizzle of Honey: 65

Mango Coconut Ice Pops: 66

CHAPTER SIX: **67**

Tips for Success on the OMAD Diet **67**

AMOUNT OF EXERCISE **68**

BENEFITS OF EXERCISE **69**

RAPID FAT LOSS EXERCISE **70**

WEIGHING FREQUENTLY **71**

CHAPTER SEVEN: **73**

LIFESTYLE **73**

HIDDEN FACTORS..**73**

TESTING FOR HIDDEN FACTORS..**74**

BLOOD SUGAR AND INSULIN..**76**

EMOTIONAL ISSUES RELATED TO OMAD............................**78**

INTRODUCTION

In a world inundated with quick fixes and fleeting promises of transformation, where the struggle against weight gain often feels like an endless battle, there exists a beacon of hope—a revolutionary approach that transcends the norms and challenges the status quo. Welcome to the world of OMAD.

Imagine a life where you no longer feel enslaved by the relentless cycle of diets and deprivation, where the weight of your struggles melts away, leaving behind a newfound sense of empowerment and freedom. The One Meal a Day (OMAD) diet beckons you to embark on a journey of self-discovery and transformation—one meal at a time, but OMAD is more than just a diet; it's a paradigm shift—a shift from restriction to liberation, from despair to hope, from self-doubt to unwavering confidence. It's about reclaiming control over your health and your life, forging a path towards a brighter, more vibrant future.

At its core, OMAD is a testament to the resilience of the human spirit—a reminder that no matter how daunting the challenges may seem, there's always a way forward. It's about embracing simplicity in a world of complexity, finding solace in the rhythm of one meal, one day, one moment at a time, if you've ever felt lost in the sea of fad diets and conflicting advice, if you've ever yearned for a solution that speaks to your soul as much as it does to your body, then take heart, for OMAD offers a sanctuary where you can rewrite your story, where every bite becomes a testament to your strength and resilience, where each meal is not just sustenance but a celebration of your journey towards health and happiness.

As you delve into the pages of this book, let yourself be guided by the promise of possibility, by the unwavering belief that within you lies the power to transform your life. Embrace the simplicity of OMAD, and let it be the catalyst for profound change—a change that extends far beyond the number on the scale, reaching into the depths of your soul.

UNDERSTAND THAT IT MIGHT TAKE SOMETIME TO ADJUST

Not surprisingly, OMAD can take some time to get used to. You've probably heard of "hanger", where you might feel angry because you're hungry. That's fasting-induced anger, and it could be a new reality for you, at least initially.

Having low blood sugar can lead to irritability and mood swings, while fasting can also lead to cortisol response(a stress hormone) which might leave you feeling anxious at first.

PICK AN OMAD STYLE THAT WORKS FOR YOUR SCHEDULE

OMAD encompasses several styles of eating. In some you'll fast during certain times daily and in others, you'll fast for one or two days per week.

The 16:8

This is where you'll only eat during eight hours per day and fast for the other 16 hours. This style might work well for parents on the go.

For example: You're up early with the kids, and amid the morning rush to get them to school and yourself to work, you skip breakfast. Soon, it's 10 a.m. and you're ready for food. At the end of the day, you're having dinner with your kids by 5:30 p.m. so they can make it to bed on time.

"Without realizing it you are already conforming to the 16:8 method of fasting — only consuming food within an eight-hour window.

The 16:8 method might also be good for gym-goers and people who have demanding work schedules.

Twice-A-Week Method Or Alternate-Day Fasting.

In both of these methods, you'll eat normally for several days per week and then only eat 500 calories on certain days. For the twice-a-week method, you'll eat 500 calories on two non-consecutive days (like Mondays and Wednesdays). In the other version, you'll restrict yourself to just 500 calories every other day.

A breakfast that consists of a two-egg omelet made with a few ounces of mozzarella cheese, a slice of whole wheat toast and a cup of blueberries could be roughly 500 calories — and that's all you'd get for the day.

This style of dieting might work well for older folks who may need fewer calories anyway because they're less active. Plus, our appetites tend to diminish as we get older.

A true 24-hour fast, completed twice weekly.

This means no food, and only water for a full day.

If you're opting for one of the reduced calorie fasts, plan to pack your snacks with protein and fiber to keep you feeling full as long as possible

Safety Considerations and Precautions

Understanding the Risks:

The OMAD diet can be mentally challenging for some individuals due to its restrictive nature. Rapid weight loss or extreme caloric restriction may lead to feelings of deprivation and frustration. It's essential to be aware of the potential psychological impacts of such dietary changes.

Consulting with a Healthcare Professional:

Before embarking on the OMAD diet or any other significant dietary change, it's crucial to consult with a healthcare professional, especially if you have pre-existing medical conditions or are taking medications. A healthcare provider can offer personalized advice based on your health history and help monitor your progress to ensure safety and effectiveness.

Monitoring Nutrient Intake:

With only one meal a day, it's important to ensure that your body receives all the essential nutrients it needs for optimal health. Monitoring your nutrient intake and possibly supplementing with vitamins or minerals may be necessary to prevent deficiencies.

Avoiding Disordered Eating Patterns:

The OMAD diet may inadvertently lead to disordered eating patterns if not approached mindfully. It's essential to be aware of the signs of orthorexia nervosa or other eating disorders, such as obsession with food quality and quantity, excessive exercise, or social withdrawal.

Hydration:

Proper hydration is essential, especially during fasting periods. Dehydration can lead to fatigue, headaches, and difficulty concentrating. Be sure to drink an adequate amount of water throughout the day to stay hydrated and support overall health.

Adjusting for Individual Needs:

Everyone's body is different, and what works for one person may not work for another. It's important to customize the OMAD diet to suit your individual health conditions, dietary preferences, and lifestyle. Listen to your body's cues and make adjustments as needed to ensure a sustainable and balanced approach to eating.

How to Follow the OMAD Diet Safely

1. Gradual Transition:

- Start by gradually reducing the number of meals you consume per day. This allows your body to adjust to the new eating pattern gradually.
- Consider implementing intermittent fasting (e.g., 16:8 method) before transitioning to OMAD to help your body adapt to fasting periods.

2. Adequate Caloric Intake:

- Ensure that your one meal a day provides enough calories to meet your body's energy needs.
- Focus on nutrient-dense foods to maximize the nutritional value of your meal.

3. Balanced Nutrition:

- Include a variety of food groups in your OMAD meal to ensure you get all the essential nutrients your body needs.
- Prioritize lean proteins, healthy fats, complex carbohydrates, and plenty of fruits and vegetables.

4. Hydration:

- Drink plenty of water throughout the day, especially during fasting periods, to stay hydrated.

- Avoid excessive consumption of caffeinated or sugary beverages, as they can disrupt hydration levels.

5. Listen to Your Body:

- Pay attention to hunger and fullness cues. Eat until you feel satisfied, but not overly full.

- If you experience extreme hunger or discomfort, consider adjusting your meal timing or portion sizes.

6. Monitor Physical and Mental Well-being:

- Keep track of your physical and mental health while following the OMAD diet.

- Watch for signs of fatigue, dizziness, weakness, mood swings, or changes in sleep patterns, which could indicate that the diet is not suitable for you.

7. Consider Professional Guidance:

- Consult with a healthcare professional or registered dietitian before starting the OMAD diet, especially if you have underlying health conditions or concerns.

- A healthcare provider can offer personalized advice and help monitor your progress to ensure safety and effectiveness.

8. Flexibility and Adaptability:

- Be flexible with your OMAD schedule and meal choices to accommodate social occasions, travel, or special events.

- Remember that the OMAD diet should enhance your overall well-being, not become a source of stress or rigidity.

9. Regular Evaluation:

- Periodically assess how the OMAD diet is affecting your health, energy levels, and overall satisfaction.

- Adjust your approach as needed to ensure a sustainable and balanced eating pattern.

CHAPTER ONE

Getting Started with the OMAD Diet

Calculating Your Caloric Needs

1. Determine Your Basal Metabolic Rate (BMR):

- Your Basal Metabolic Rate (BMR) represents the number of calories your body needs to maintain basic physiological functions at rest, such as breathing, circulation, and cell production.

- Various formulas can estimate your BMR, with the Harris-Benedict equation being one commonly used method. The equation takes into account your age, gender, weight, and height.

- For example, the Harris-Benedict equation for men is: BMR = 88.362 + (13.397 × weight in kg) + (4.799 × height in cm) - (5.677 × age in years)

- And for women: BMR = 447.593 + (9.247 × weight in kg) + (3.098 × height in cm) - (4.330 × age in years)

2. Factor in Activity Level:

- Once you've calculated your BMR, you need to adjust it based on your activity level. This accounts for the calories you burn through daily activities and exercise.

- Use a multiplier based on your activity level:

    - Sedentary (little to no exercise): BMR × 1.2

    - Lightly active (light exercise/sports 1-3 days/week): BMR × 1.375

    - Moderately active (moderate exercise/sports 3-5 days/week): BMR × 1.55

    - Very active (hard exercise/sports 6-7 days a week): BMR × 1.725

    - Extra active (very hard exercise/sports & physical job or training twice a day): BMR × 1.9

3. Adjust for Weight Goals:

- If your goal is weight loss, you'll need to create a calorie deficit by consuming fewer calories than your total energy expenditure (TEE). A deficit of 500-1000 calories per day typically results in a safe and sustainable weight loss of 1-2 pounds per week.

- If your goal is weight maintenance or muscle gain, adjust your calorie intake accordingly. Aim to consume slightly more or fewer calories than your TEE, depending on your specific goals.

4. Monitor and Adjust:

- Keep track of your food intake and monitor your progress regularly. Use a food diary or mobile app to log your meals and calculate your daily calorie intake.

- Pay attention to how your body responds to your OMAD meal plan. Adjust your calorie intake and meal composition as needed to achieve your desired outcomes.

- Consult with a healthcare professional or registered dietitian for personalized guidance and support, especially if you have specific health concerns or dietary restrictions.

Choosing the Right Foods for Your OMAD Meals

1. Prioritize Nutrient-Dense Foods:

- Focus on incorporating whole, minimally processed foods that are rich in essential nutrients such as vitamins, minerals, fiber, and antioxidants.

- Choose a variety of colorful fruits and vegetables to ensure you're getting a wide range of vitamins and minerals.

2. Include Lean Proteins:

- Protein is essential for muscle repair, growth, and overall health. Include lean sources of protein such as poultry, fish, tofu, tempeh, legumes, and low-fat dairy products in your OMAD meals.

- Aim to include a palm-sized portion of protein in your meal to help keep you feeling full and satisfied.

3. Incorporate Healthy Fats:

- Healthy fats are important for hormone production, brain function, and satiety. Include sources of unsaturated fats such as avocados, nuts, seeds, olive oil, and fatty fish like salmon or mackerel in your OMAD meals.

- Use these fats as dressings, toppings, or cooking oils to add flavor and richness to your meals.

4. Choose Complex Carbohydrates:

- Opt for complex carbohydrates that provide sustained energy and are rich in fiber, such as whole grains, legumes, sweet potatoes, and quinoa.

- These carbohydrates are digested more slowly, helping to stabilize blood sugar levels and keep you feeling full for longer periods.

5. Limit Added Sugars and Processed Foods:

- Minimize your intake of added sugars, refined grains, and processed foods, as they provide empty calories and may lead to blood sugar spikes and crashes.

- Instead, choose whole, unprocessed foods whenever possible and sweeten foods naturally with fruits or small amounts of honey or maple syrup.

6. Pay Attention to Portion Sizes:

- While following the OMAD diet, it's important to be mindful of portion sizes to avoid overeating during your single meal.

- Use smaller plates or bowls to help control portion sizes visually, and listen to your body's hunger and satiety cues to determine when you've had enough.

7. Stay Hydrated:

- Don't forget to hydrate adequately throughout the day, even during fasting periods. Water is essential for digestion, metabolism, and overall health.

- Consider incorporating hydrating foods like cucumbers, watermelon, and leafy greens into your OMAD meal to help meet your fluid needs.

8. Experiment and Enjoy:

- Get creative with your OMAD meals and experiment with different flavors, textures, and cuisines to keep things interesting and enjoyable.

- Incorporate a variety of foods from different food groups to ensure a well-rounded and satisfying meal.

Meal Planning and Preparation Tips

1. Set Aside Dedicated Time:

- Schedule a specific time each week for meal planning and preparation. This could be on the weekend or a day when you have the most free time.

- Dedicate a few hours to plan your meals, create a shopping list, and prepare ingredients in advance.

2. Plan Balanced Meals:

- Aim to include a balance of protein, healthy fats, complex carbohydrates, and plenty of vegetables in your OMAD meal.

- Use the "plate method" as a guide: fill half your plate with non-starchy vegetables, one-quarter with lean protein, and one-quarter with whole grains or starchy vegetables.

3. Batch Cooking:

- Prepare larger batches of staple ingredients such as grains, proteins, and vegetables that can be used in multiple meals throughout the week.

- Cook grains like quinoa, brown rice, or farro in bulk and portion them out for easy meal assembly.

- Roast a variety of vegetables on a sheet pan and store them in the refrigerator to add to salads, bowls, or wraps.

4. Use Time-Saving Cooking Methods:

- Utilize time-saving cooking methods such as pressure cooking, slow cooking, or sheet pan roasting to prepare meals efficiently.

- Invest in kitchen appliances like an Instant Pot or slow cooker to simplify meal preparation and save time.

5. Pre-Portion Ingredients:

- Pre-portion ingredients for your OMAD meals to streamline the cooking process and prevent overeating.

- Measure out portions of proteins, grains, and vegetables in advance and store them in separate containers for easy access when assembling meals.

6. Plan for Leftovers:

- Embrace leftovers as a convenient way to save time and reduce food waste. Cook extra portions of your OMAD meal to enjoy as leftovers for future meals.

- Store leftovers in individual containers for easy grab-and-go meals or quick reheating.

7. Incorporate Convenience Foods:

- Don't hesitate to use convenience foods like pre-cut vegetables, canned beans, or pre-cooked proteins to save time during meal preparation.

- Look for healthy convenience options with minimal added ingredients or preservatives.

8. Stay Organized:

- Keep your kitchen organized and stocked with essential ingredients and tools for meal preparation.

- Use clear containers for storing prepped ingredients and leftovers to easily see what you have on hand.

9. Be Flexible:

- Remain flexible with your meal planning and preparation approach. Allow room for spontaneity and adjust your plan as needed based on your schedule and preferences.

- Don't stress if your meal plan doesn't go exactly as planned. Focus on making healthy choices and enjoy the process of preparing nourishing meals.

Grocery Shopping for the OMAD Diet

1. Make a Detailed Shopping List:

- Before heading to the grocery store, create a detailed shopping list based on your planned OMAD meals for the week.

- Include a variety of foods from different food groups, such as lean proteins, healthy fats, complex carbohydrates, and plenty of fruits and vegetables.

2. Stock Up on Staple Ingredients:

- Ensure you have a supply of staple ingredients that can be used in multiple OMAD meals, such as:

  - Protein sources: Chicken breast, turkey, lean beef, fish, tofu, tempeh, eggs, beans, lentils.

  - Whole grains: Brown rice, quinoa, oats, barley, whole wheat pasta.

  - Healthy fats: Avocado, nuts, seeds, olive oil, coconut oil.

  - Vegetables: Leafy greens, bell peppers, tomatoes, cucumbers, carrots, broccoli, cauliflower.

  - Fruits: Berries, apples, oranges, bananas, grapes, melons.

  - Herbs and spices: Garlic, ginger, basil, cilantro, oregano, cumin, turmeric.

3. Choose Fresh, Seasonal Produce:

- Opt for fresh, seasonal fruits and vegetables whenever possible to maximize flavor and nutritional value.

- Visit the produce section of the grocery store and choose a variety of colorful fruits and vegetables to incorporate into your OMAD meals.

4. Read Labels Carefully:

- When purchasing packaged foods, read labels carefully to check for added sugars, unhealthy fats, and artificial additives.

- Choose minimally processed, whole food options with simple ingredient lists and avoid highly processed or overly refined products.

5. Consider Frozen and Canned Options:

- Don't overlook frozen and canned options, especially for fruits, vegetables, and proteins.

- Frozen fruits and vegetables are convenient and often retain their nutritional value, while canned beans and fish can be convenient protein sources.

6. Plan for Beverages and Snacks:

- Include beverages and snacks on your shopping list to ensure you have options that align with your OMAD diet goals.

- Choose hydrating beverages such as water, herbal tea, and sparkling water, and opt for healthy snacks like nuts, seeds, Greek yogurt, and fresh fruit.

7. Shop with a Budget in Mind:

- Plan your grocery shopping trip with a budget in mind to avoid overspending.

- Look for sales, discounts, and coupons to save money on staple items and buy in bulk when possible to maximize savings.

8. Be Mindful of Portion Sizes:

- When purchasing items in bulk or larger packages, be mindful of portion sizes to prevent food waste and overconsumption.

- Consider portioning out larger packages into smaller containers or bags to help control portions and avoid overeating.

9. Stay Organized and Efficient:

- Organize your shopping list by categories (e.g., produce, dairy, proteins) to streamline your shopping trip and ensure you don't forget any items.

- Consider shopping online or using grocery delivery services for added convenience and efficiency, especially if you have a busy schedule.

Apple Cinnamon Overnight Oats:

Prep Time: 5 minutes Chill Time: **Overnight Servings:** 2

Ingredients:

- 1 cup old-fashioned oats
- 1 cup almond milk (or any milk of choice)
- 1 medium apple, diced
- 2 tablespoons maple syrup or honey
- 1 teaspoon ground cinnamon
- 1/4 teaspoon vanilla extract
- Pinch of salt
- Optional toppings: sliced almonds, chopped walnuts, additional diced apple, Greek yogurt

Instructions:

1. In a mixing bowl or jar, combine the old-fashioned oats, almond milk, diced apple, maple syrup or honey, ground cinnamon, vanilla extract, and a pinch of salt.
2. Stir well to combine all ingredients.
3. Cover the bowl or jar with a lid or plastic wrap and refrigerate overnight, or for at least 4 hours, to allow the oats to soften and absorb the liquid.
4. Before serving, give the overnight oats a good stir.
5. If desired, top with sliced almonds, chopped walnuts, additional diced apple, or a dollop of Greek yogurt.
6. Enjoy your delicious and nutritious Apple Cinnamon Overnight Oats!

Nutritional Values (Approximate): Calories: 250-300 kcal | Protein: 5-7 grams | Fat: 5-7 grams | Carbohydrates: 45-50 grams | Fiber: 7-9 grams | Sugars: 15-20 grams

Vegetable Breakfast Skillet:

Prep Time: 10 minutes   **Cook Time:** 15 minutes   **Servings:** 2

Ingredients:

- 1 tablespoon olive oil
- 1 small onion, diced
- 1 bell pepper, diced
- 1 zucchini, diced
- 1 cup cherry tomatoes, halved
- 2 cloves garlic, minced
- 4 large eggs
- Salt and pepper to taste
- Fresh parsley or basil for garnish (optional)
- Grated cheese (optional)

Instructions:

1. Heat olive oil in a large skillet over medium heat.
2. Add diced onion and bell pepper to the skillet. Cook for 3-4 minutes until softened.
3. Add diced zucchini and minced garlic to the skillet. Cook for an additional 3-4 minutes until vegetables are tender.
4. Add cherry tomatoes to the skillet and cook for 2-3 minutes until they start to soften.
5. Create small wells in the vegetable mixture and crack eggs into each well.
6. Season eggs with salt and pepper to taste.
7. Cover the skillet and cook for 5-7 minutes, or until eggs are cooked to your desired doneness.
8. Sprinkle with grated cheese if desired, and garnish with fresh parsley or basil.
9. Serve hot, directly from the skillet.

Nutritional Values (Approximate): Calories: 250-300 kcal | Protein: 15-18 grams | Fat: 15-18 grams | Carbohydrates: 10-12 grams | Fiber: 3-5 grams | Sugars: 5-7 grams

Banana Oat Pancakes:

Prep Time: 10 minutes   **Cook Time:** 10 minutes   **Servings:** 2 (6 small pancakes)

Ingredients:

- 1 ripe banana
- 1 cup rolled oats
- 1/2 cup almond milk (or any milk of choice)
- 1 egg
- 1 teaspoon baking powder
- 1/2 teaspoon ground cinnamon
- 1/4 teaspoon vanilla extract
- Pinch of salt
- Butter or oil for cooking

Instructions:

1. In a blender or food processor, combine the ripe banana, rolled oats, almond milk, egg, baking powder, ground cinnamon, vanilla extract, and a pinch of salt. Blend until smooth.
2. Heat a non-stick skillet or griddle over medium heat and lightly grease with butter or oil.
3. Pour small amounts of the pancake batter onto the skillet to form pancakes.
4. Cook for 2-3 minutes on one side, until bubbles form on the surface of the pancake.
5. Flip the pancakes and cook for an additional 1-2 minutes on the other side, until golden brown and cooked through.
6. Repeat with the remaining batter.
7. Serve hot with your favorite toppings such as sliced bananas, berries, maple syrup, or Greek yogurt.

Nutritional Values (Approximate): Calories: 200-250 kcal | Protein: 8-10 grams | Fat: 5-7 grams | Carbohydrates: 30-35 grams | Fiber: 4-6 grams | Sugars: 10-12 grams

Spinach and Mushroom Frittata:

Prep Time: 10 minutes   **Cook Time:** 20 minutes   **Servings:** 4

Ingredients:

- 6 large eggs
- 1/4 cup milk (or dairy-free milk alternative)
- 1 tablespoon olive oil
- 1 small onion, diced
- 2 cups fresh spinach leaves, chopped
- 1 cup mushrooms, sliced
- 2 cloves garlic, minced
- Salt and pepper to taste
- 1/4 cup grated cheese (optional)
- Fresh parsley for garnish (optional)

Instructions:

1. Preheat the oven to 350°F (175°C).
2. In a mixing bowl, whisk together eggs and milk until well combined. Season with salt and pepper.
3. Heat olive oil in an oven-safe skillet over medium heat.
4. Add diced onion and sliced mushrooms to the skillet. Cook for 5-7 minutes until mushrooms are golden brown and onions are softened.
5. Add minced garlic and chopped spinach to the skillet. Cook for an additional 2-3 minutes until spinach is wilted.
6. Pour the egg mixture evenly over the vegetables in the skillet. Stir gently to distribute the vegetables.
7. Sprinkle grated cheese evenly over the top of the frittata, if using.
8. Transfer the skillet to the preheated oven and bake for 15-20 minutes, or until the frittata is set in the center and lightly golden on top.
9. Remove from the oven and let it cool slightly before slicing.
10. Garnish with fresh parsley, if desired, and serve warm or at room temperature.

Nutritional Values (Approximate): Calories: 150-200 kcal | Protein: 10-12 grams | Fat: 10-12 grams | Carbohydrates: 5-7 grams | Fiber: 1-2 grams | Sugars: 2-3 grams

Peanut Butter and Banana Smoothie:

Prep Time: 5 minutes   **Servings:** 2

Ingredients:

- 2 ripe bananas, peeled and sliced
- 2 tablespoons peanut butter
- 1 cup milk (or dairy-free milk alternative)
- 1/2 cup Greek yogurt
- 1 tablespoon honey or maple syrup (optional)
- 1/2 teaspoon vanilla extract
- 4-6 ice cubes

Instructions:

1. In a blender, combine sliced bananas, peanut butter, milk, Greek yogurt, honey or maple syrup (if using), vanilla extract, and ice cubes.
2. Blend on high speed until smooth and creamy.
3. Taste and adjust sweetness if necessary by adding more honey or maple syrup.
4. Pour into glasses and serve immediately.

Nutritional Values (Approximate): Calories: 300-350 kcal | Protein: 12-15 grams | Fat: 15-18 grams | Carbohydrates: 30-35 grams | Fiber: 4-6 grams | Sugars: 20-25 grams

Prep Time: 10 minutes   **Cook Time:** 20 minutes   **Servings:** 2

Ingredients:

- 2 medium sweet potatoes, peeled and diced
- 2 tablespoons olive oil
- 1 small onion, diced
- 1 bell pepper, diced
- 2 cloves garlic, minced
- 1 teaspoon paprika
- 1/2 teaspoon ground cumin
- Salt and pepper to taste
- 4 large eggs
- Fresh parsley or cilantro for garnish (optional)
- Hot sauce for serving (optional)

Instructions:

1. Heat olive oil in a large skillet over medium heat.
2. Add diced sweet potatoes to the skillet. Cook for 8-10 minutes, stirring occasionally, until sweet potatoes are tender and lightly browned.
3. Add diced onion, bell pepper, and minced garlic to the skillet. Cook for an additional 5-7 minutes until vegetables are softened.
4. Stir in paprika, ground cumin, salt, and pepper. Cook for 1-2 minutes until fragrant.
5. Create small wells in the sweet potato mixture and crack eggs into each well.
6. Cover the skillet and cook for 4-5 minutes, or until eggs are cooked to your desired doneness.
7. Remove from heat and garnish with fresh parsley or cilantro, if desired.
8. Serve hot, directly from the skillet, with hot sauce on the side if desired.

Nutritional Values (Approximate): Calories: 300-350 kcal | Protein: 10-12 grams | Fat: 15-18 grams | Carbohydrates: 30-35 grams | Fiber: 5-7 grams | Sugars: 8-10 grams

Scrambled Eggs with Spinach and Tomatoes:

Prep Time: 5 minutes   **Cook Time:** 10 minutes   **Servings:** 2

Ingredients:

- 4 large eggs
- 2 cups fresh spinach leaves, chopped
- 1 cup cherry tomatoes, halved
- 2 tablespoons olive oil
- 2 cloves garlic, minced
- Salt and pepper to taste
- Feta cheese for garnish (optional)
- Fresh herbs for garnish (optional)

Instructions:

1. In a bowl, whisk the eggs until well beaten. Set aside.
2. Heat olive oil in a skillet over medium heat.
3. Add minced garlic to the skillet and cook for 1 minute until fragrant.
4. Add chopped spinach to the skillet and cook for 2-3 minutes until wilted.
5. Add halved cherry tomatoes to the skillet and cook for another 2-3 minutes until softened.
6. Pour the beaten eggs into the skillet with the spinach and tomatoes.
7. Season with salt and pepper to taste.
8. Cook, stirring gently, until the eggs are scrambled and cooked to your desired consistency.
9. Remove from heat and garnish with crumbled feta cheese and fresh herbs if desired.
10. Serve hot.

Nutritional Values (Approximate): Calories: 250-300 kcal | Protein: 15-18 grams | Fat: 18-20 grams | Carbohydrates: 8-10 grams | Fiber: 2-3 grams | Sugars: 2-3 grams

Greek Yogurt with Honey and Mixed Berries:

Prep Time: 5 minutes   **Servings:** 2

Ingredients:

- 1 cup Greek yogurt
- 2 tablespoons honey
- 1 cup mixed berries (such as strawberries, blueberries, raspberries)
- 2 tablespoons chopped nuts (such as almonds, walnuts, or pecans) (optional)

Instructions:

1. Divide Greek yogurt evenly between two serving bowls.
2. Drizzle 1 tablespoon of honey over each serving of yogurt.
3. Top with mixed berries and chopped nuts, if desired.
4. Serve immediately.

Nutritional Values (Approximate): Calories: 200-250 kcal | Protein: 10-12 grams | Fat: 5-7 grams | Carbohydrates: 30-35 grams | Fiber: 3-5 grams | Sugars: 25-30 grams

Quinoa Breakfast Bowl with Almond Milk and Berries:

Prep Time: 5 minutes   **Cook Time:** 15 minutes   **Servings:** 2

Ingredients:

- 1/2 cup quinoa, rinsed
- 1 cup almond milk (or any milk of choice)
- 1/2 cup mixed berries (such as strawberries, blueberries, and raspberries)
- 2 tablespoons sliced almonds
- 1 tablespoon honey or maple syrup (optional)

Instructions:

1. In a saucepan, combine quinoa and almond milk. Bring to a boil, then reduce heat to low, cover, and simmer for 15 minutes or until quinoa is cooked and liquid is absorbed.
2. Divide the cooked quinoa into bowls.

3. Top with mixed berries and sliced almonds.

4. Drizzle with honey or maple syrup if desired.

5. Serve warm.

Nutritional Values (Approximate): Calories: 250-300 kcal | Protein: 8-10 grams | Fat: 5-7 grams | Carbohydrates: 40-45 grams | Fiber: 6-8 grams | Sugars: 8-10 grams

Avocado Toast with Poached Egg:

Prep Time: 5 minutes   **Cook Time:** 5 minutes   **Servings:** 2

Ingredients:

- 2 slices whole grain bread

- 1 ripe avocado

- 2 large eggs

- Salt and pepper to taste

- Red pepper flakes for garnish (optional)

- Fresh herbs for garnish (such as cilantro or parsley) (optional)

Instructions:

1. Toast the slices of whole grain bread until golden brown.

2. While the bread is toasting, cut the avocado in half, remove the pit, and scoop the flesh into a bowl. Mash the avocado with a fork until smooth.

3. Poach the eggs: Bring a pot of water to a gentle simmer. Crack each egg into a small bowl or ramekin. Create a gentle whirlpool in the simmering water with a spoon and carefully slide the eggs, one at a time, into the center of the whirlpool. Cook for 3-4 minutes for a soft yolk or longer for a firmer yolk.

4. Spread the mashed avocado evenly onto the toasted bread slices.

5. Carefully remove the poached eggs from the water using a slotted spoon and place one egg on top of each slice of avocado toast.

6. Season with salt, pepper, and red pepper flakes if desired.

7. Garnish with fresh herbs if desired.

8. Serve immediately.

Nutritional Values (Approximate): Calories: 250-300 kcal | Protein: 10-12 grams | Fat: 15-18 grams | Carbohydrates: 20-25 grams | Fiber: 7-9 grams | Sugars: 1-2 grams

CHAPTER THREE

Grilled Chicken Salad:

Prep Time: 15 minutes   **Cook Time:** 10 minutes   **Servings:** 2

Ingredients:

- 2 boneless, skinless chicken breasts
- 4 cups mixed greens (such as lettuce, spinach, arugula)
- 1 cup cherry tomatoes, halved
- 1/2 cucumber, sliced
- 1/4 red onion, thinly sliced
- 1/4 cup crumbled feta cheese
- 2 tablespoons olive oil
- 1 tablespoon balsamic vinegar
- Salt and pepper to taste

Instructions:

1. Preheat grill to medium-high heat.
2. Season chicken breasts with salt and pepper.
3. Grill chicken for 4-5 minutes per side, or until cooked through and no longer pink in the center.
4. In a large bowl, combine mixed greens, cherry tomatoes, cucumber, red onion, and feta cheese.
5. In a small bowl, whisk together olive oil and balsamic vinegar to make the dressing.
6. Slice grilled chicken and add to the salad.
7. Drizzle dressing over the salad and toss to combine.
8. Divide salad between plates and serve.

Nutritional Values (Approximate): Calories: 300-350 kcal Protein: 30-35 grams Fat: 15-18 grams Carbohydrates: 10-12 grams Fiber: 3-5 grams Sugars: 5-7 grams

Quinoa Stuffed Bell Peppers:

Prep Time: 20 minutes   **Cook Time:** 30 minutes   **Servings:** 4

Ingredients:

- 4 bell peppers, any color
- 1 cup quinoa, rinsed
- 2 cups vegetable broth or water
- 1 can (15 oz) black beans, rinsed and drained
- 1 cup corn kernels
- 1 cup diced tomatoes
- 1/2 cup diced red onion
- 1/4 cup chopped fresh cilantro
- 1 teaspoon ground cumin
- 1/2 teaspoon chili powder
- Salt and pepper to taste
- 1/2 cup shredded cheese (optional)

Instructions:

1. Preheat oven to 375°F (190°C).
2. Cut the tops off the bell peppers and remove the seeds and membranes.
3. In a medium saucepan, combine quinoa and vegetable broth. Bring to a boil, then reduce heat to low, cover, and simmer for 15 minutes, or until quinoa is cooked and liquid is absorbed.
4. In a large bowl, combine cooked quinoa, black beans, corn, diced tomatoes, red onion, cilantro, cumin, chili powder, salt, and pepper. Mix well.
5. Stuff each bell pepper with the quinoa mixture.
6. Place stuffed peppers in a baking dish. If using cheese, sprinkle it over the tops of the peppers.
7. Cover the baking dish with foil and bake for 25-30 minutes, or until peppers are tender.
8. Remove foil and bake for an additional 5 minutes, or until cheese is melted and bubbly (if using).
9. Serve hot.

Nutritional Values (Approximate): Calories: 300-350 kcal | Protein: 10-12 grams | Fat: 5-7 grams | Carbohydrates: 55-60 grams | Fiber: 10-12 grams | Sugars: 5-7 grams

Salmon and Asparagus Foil Pack:

Prep Time: 10 minutes   **Cook Time:** 20 minutes   **Servings:** 2

Ingredients:

- 2 salmon fillets
- 1 bunch asparagus, trimmed
- 1 lemon, thinly sliced
- 2 tablespoons olive oil
- 2 cloves garlic, minced
- Salt and pepper to taste
- Fresh dill for garnish (optional)

Instructions:

1. Preheat oven to 400°F (200°C).
2. Place each salmon fillet on a large piece of foil.
3. Arrange asparagus spears around each salmon fillet.
4. Top salmon and asparagus with lemon slices and minced garlic.
5. Drizzle olive oil over salmon and asparagus. Season with salt and pepper.
6. Fold the edges of the foil to create a packet, sealing tightly.
7. Place foil packets on a baking sheet and bake for 15-20 minutes, or until salmon is cooked through and asparagus is tender.
8. Carefully open foil packets and transfer salmon and asparagus to plates.
9. Garnish with fresh dill, if desired, and serve hot.

Nutritional Values (Approximate): Calories: 350-400 kcal | Protein: 30-35 grams | Fat: 20-25 grams | Carbohydrates: 10-12 grams | Fiber: 5-7 grams | Sugars: 3-5 grams

Baked Lemon Herb Chicken:

Prep Time: 10 minutes   **Cook Time:** 25 minutes   **Servings:** 4

Ingredients:

- 4 boneless, skinless chicken breasts
- 2 tablespoons olive oil
- 2 tablespoons fresh lemon juice
- 2 cloves garlic, minced
- 1 teaspoon dried thyme
- 1 teaspoon dried rosemary
- 1 teaspoon dried oregano
- Salt and pepper to taste
- Lemon slices for garnish (optional)
- Fresh parsley for garnish (optional)

Instructions:

1. Preheat oven to 400°F (200°C).
2. In a small bowl, whisk together olive oil, lemon juice, minced garlic, dried thyme, dried rosemary, dried oregano, salt, and pepper.
3. Place chicken breasts in a baking dish. Pour the lemon herb marinade over the chicken, making sure each piece is coated evenly.
4. Arrange lemon slices on top of the chicken breasts, if desired.
5. Bake for 20-25 minutes, or until chicken is cooked through and juices run clear.
6. Garnish with fresh parsley, if desired, and serve hot.

Nutritional Values (Approximate): Calories: 250-300 kcal | Protein: 30-35 grams | Fat: 10-12 grams | Carbohydrates: 2-4 grams | Fiber: 1-2 grams | Sugars: 1 gram

Prep Time: 15 minutes   **Cook Time:** 15 minutes   **Servings:** 4

Ingredients:

- 1 lb beef sirloin or flank steak, thinly sliced
- 2 tablespoons soy sauce
- 1 tablespoon oyster sauce
- 1 tablespoon sesame oil
- 2 cloves garlic, minced
- 1 teaspoon grated ginger
- 1 tablespoon cornstarch
- 2 tablespoons vegetable oil
- 4 cups broccoli florets
- 1 red bell pepper, thinly sliced
- 1 yellow bell pepper, thinly sliced
- Cooked rice or quinoa, for serving
- Sesame seeds for garnish (optional)
- Sliced green onions for garnish (optional)

Instructions:

1. In a bowl, combine thinly sliced beef with soy sauce, oyster sauce, sesame oil, minced garlic, grated ginger, and cornstarch. Let marinate for at least 10 minutes.

2. Heat vegetable oil in a large skillet or wok over medium-high heat.

3. Add marinated beef to the skillet and stir-fry for 2-3 minutes, or until beef is browned and cooked through. Remove beef from skillet and set aside.

4. In the same skillet, add broccoli florets and sliced bell peppers. Stir-fry for 3-4 minutes, or until vegetables are tender-crisp.

5. Return cooked beef to the skillet and toss with the vegetables.

6. Serve hot over cooked rice or quinoa.

7. Garnish with sesame seeds and sliced green onions, if desired.

Nutritional Values (Approximate): Calories: 300-350 kcal | Protein: 25-30 grams | Fat: 15-18 grams | Carbohydrates: 15-20 grams | Fiber: 5-7 grams | Sugars: 5-7 grams

Shrimp and Zucchini Noodles:

Prep Time: 10 minutes   **Cook Time:** 10 minutes   **Servings:** 2

Ingredients:

- 8 oz shrimp, peeled and deveined
- 2 medium zucchini, spiralized into noodles
- 2 cloves garlic, minced
- 1 tablespoon olive oil
- 1/2 teaspoon red pepper flakes
- Salt and pepper to taste
- Fresh parsley for garnish (optional)
- Lemon wedges for serving

Instructions:

1. Heat olive oil in a large skillet over medium heat.
2. Add minced garlic and red pepper flakes to the skillet. Cook for 1 minute until fragrant.
3. Add shrimp to the skillet and cook for 2-3 minutes on each side, until pink and cooked through. Season with salt and pepper.
4. Push the shrimp to one side of the skillet and add zucchini noodles. Cook for 2-3 minutes, tossing occasionally, until noodles are tender but still slightly crisp.
5. Serve shrimp and zucchini noodles hot, garnished with fresh parsley and lemon wedges.

Nutritional Values (Approximate): Calories: 250-300 kcal | Protein: 25-30 grams | Fat: 10-12 grams | Carbohydrates: 10-12 grams | Fiber: 3-5 grams | Sugars: 5-7 grams

Lentil Soup with Vegetables:

Prep Time: 15 minutes   **Cook Time:** 30 minutes   **Servings:** 4

Ingredients:

- 1 cup dried lentils, rinsed
- 4 cups vegetable broth
- 1 onion, diced
- 2 carrots, diced
- 2 celery stalks, diced
- 2 cloves garlic, minced
- 1 teaspoon dried thyme
- 1 teaspoon dried oregano
- Salt and pepper to taste
- Fresh parsley for garnish (optional)

Instructions:

1. In a large pot, heat olive oil over medium heat.
2. Add diced onion, carrots, and celery to the pot. Cook for 5-7 minutes, until vegetables are softened.
3. Add minced garlic, dried thyme, and dried oregano to the pot. Cook for 1 minute until fragrant.
4. Add dried lentils and vegetable broth to the pot. Bring to a boil, then reduce heat and simmer for 20-25 minutes, until lentils are tender.
5. Season with salt and pepper to taste.
6. Serve hot, garnished with fresh parsley if desired.

Nutritional Values (Approximate): Calories: 200-250 kcal | Protein: 15-18 grams | Fat: 1-2 grams | Carbohydrates: 35-40 grams | Fiber: 15-18 grams | Sugars: 5-7 grams

Prep Time: 15 minutes   **Cook Time:** 10 minutes   **Servings:** 2

Ingredients:

- 1 lb ground turkey
- 2 tablespoons olive oil
- 2 cloves garlic, minced
- 1 small onion, diced
- 1 bell pepper, diced
- 1/2 cup mushrooms, diced
- 2 tablespoons soy sauce
- 1 tablespoon hoisin sauce
- 1 teaspoon sesame oil
- Salt and pepper to taste
- 1 avocado, sliced
- Lettuce leaves, for wrapping
- Sriracha sauce for serving (optional)

Instructions:

1. Heat olive oil in a large skillet over medium heat.
2. Add minced garlic and diced onion to the skillet. Cook for 2-3 minutes until softened.
3. Add ground turkey to the skillet. Cook, breaking it apart with a spoon, until browned and cooked through.
4. Add diced bell pepper and mushrooms to the skillet. Cook for an additional 3-4 minutes until vegetables are tender.
5. Stir in soy sauce, hoisin sauce, and sesame oil. Season with salt and pepper to taste.
6. Remove skillet from heat and assemble lettuce wraps by spooning turkey mixture onto lettuce leaves.
7. Top with sliced avocado and drizzle with sriracha sauce if desired.
8. Serve immediately.

Nutritional Values (Approximate): Calories: 300-350 kcal | Protein: 25-30 grams | Fat: 15-18 grams | Carbohydrates: 15-20 grams | Fiber: 5-7 grams | Sugars: 5-7 grams

Cauliflower Fried Rice with Tofu:

Prep Time: 15 minutes   **Cook Time:** 15 minutes   **Servings:** 2

Ingredients:

- 1 small head cauliflower, grated or riced
- 1 tablespoon sesame oil
- 1 block firm tofu, diced
- 2 cloves garlic, minced
- 1 small onion, diced
- 1 cup mixed vegetables (such as peas, carrots, corn)
- 2 tablespoons soy sauce
- 1 tablespoon rice vinegar
- 2 green onions, thinly sliced
- Sesame seeds for garnish (optional)

Instructions:

1. Heat sesame oil in a large skillet or wok over medium heat.
2. Add diced tofu to the skillet and cook until golden brown and crispy, about 5-7 minutes. Remove tofu from skillet and set aside.
3. In the same skillet, add minced garlic and diced onion. Cook for 2-3 minutes until softened.
4. Add mixed vegetables to the skillet and cook for an additional 3-4 minutes until tender.
5. Stir in grated cauliflower, soy sauce, and rice vinegar. Cook for 3-4 minutes, stirring occasionally.
6. Return cooked tofu to the skillet and toss to combine with the cauliflower rice.
7. Garnish with sliced green onions and sesame seeds, if desired.
8. Serve hot.

Nutritional Values (Approximate): Calories: 250-300 kcal | Protein: 20-25 grams | Fat: 10-12 grams | Carbohydrates: 20-25 grams | Fiber: 7-10 grams | Sugars: 5-7 grams

Veggie Frittata with Spinach and Feta:

Prep Time: 10 minutes   **Cook Time:** 20 minutes   **Servings:** 4

Ingredients:

- 8 large eggs
- 1/4 cup milk (or dairy-free milk alternative)
- 1 tablespoon olive oil
- 2 cups fresh spinach leaves
- 1/2 cup diced bell pepper
- 1/4 cup diced red onion
- 1/4 cup crumbled feta cheese
- Salt and pepper to taste
- Fresh parsley for garnish (optional)

Instructions:

1. Preheat the oven to 350°F (175°C).
2. In a mixing bowl, whisk together eggs and milk until well combined. Season with salt and pepper.
3. Heat olive oil in an oven-safe skillet over medium heat.
4. Add diced bell pepper and red onion to the skillet. Cook for 2-3 minutes until softened.
5. Add fresh spinach leaves to the skillet and cook for another 1-2 minutes until wilted.
6. Pour the egg mixture over the vegetables in the skillet. Stir gently to distribute the vegetables evenly.
7. Sprinkle crumbled feta cheese over the top of the frittata.
8. Transfer the skillet to the preheated oven and bake for 15-20 minutes, or until the frittata is set in the center and lightly golden on top.
9. Remove from the oven and let it cool slightly before slicing.
10. Garnish with fresh parsley, if desired, and serve warm or at room temperature.

Nutritional Values (Approximate): Calories: 200-250 kcal | Protein: 15-18 grams | Fat: 12-15 grams | Carbohydrates: 5-7 grams | Fiber: 1-2 grams | Sugars: 2-3 grams

Grilled Salmon with Roasted Vegetables:

Prep Time: 15 minutes   **Cook Time:** 25 minutes   **Servings:** 4

Ingredients:

- 4 salmon fillets (about 6 ounces each), skin-on
- 2 tablespoons olive oil
- 1 teaspoon lemon zest
- 2 tablespoons lemon juice
- 2 cloves garlic, minced
- 1 teaspoon dried oregano
- Salt and black pepper to taste
- 2 bell peppers, sliced
- 1 large zucchini, sliced
- 1 large red onion, sliced
- 1 pint cherry tomatoes
- 2 tablespoons balsamic vinegar
- Fresh parsley, chopped (for garnish)

Instructions:

1. Preheat your grill to medium-high heat.

2. In a small bowl, whisk together 1 tablespoon of olive oil, lemon zest, lemon juice, minced garlic, dried oregano, salt, and black pepper.

3. Place the salmon fillets in a shallow dish and pour the marinade over them. Make sure the fillets are evenly coated. Let them marinate for about 10 minutes while you prepare the vegetables.

4. In a large bowl, toss the sliced bell peppers, zucchini, red onion, and cherry tomatoes with the remaining olive oil and balsamic vinegar. Season with salt and black pepper to taste.

5. Spread the vegetables out in a single layer on a baking sheet lined with parchment paper.

6. Place the salmon fillets skin-side down on the preheated grill. Grill for about 4-5 minutes per side, or until the salmon is cooked through and easily flakes with a fork.

7. While the salmon is grilling, roast the vegetables in the preheated oven at 400°F (200°C) for about 20-25 minutes, or until they are tender and slightly caramelized.

8. Once the salmon and vegetables are cooked, remove them from the grill and oven.

9. Serve the grilled salmon fillets with the roasted vegetables on the side.

10. Garnish with chopped fresh parsley before serving.

Nutritional Values (Approximate): Calories: 300-350 kcal per serving | Protein: 25-30 grams | Fat: 15-20 grams | Carbohydrates: 15-20 grams | Fiber: 5-7 grams | Sugars: 8-10 grams

Cauliflower Fried Rice with Shrimp:

Prep Time: 15 minutes   **Cook Time:** 15 minutes   **Servings:** 4

Ingredients:

- 1 medium head cauliflower, grated or finely chopped
- 1 tablespoon sesame oil
- 1 onion, diced
- 2 cloves garlic, minced
- 1 cup frozen peas and carrots, thawed
- 1/2 pound shrimp, peeled and deveined
- 2 eggs, beaten
- 3 tablespoons soy sauce (or tamari for gluten-free)
- 2 green onions, chopped
- Salt and pepper to taste

Instructions:

1. Heat sesame oil in a large skillet or wok over medium heat.
2. Add diced onion and minced garlic to the skillet. Cook until fragrant and softened, about 2-3 minutes.
3. Add shrimp to the skillet and cook until pink and cooked through, about 3-4 minutes. Remove shrimp from skillet and set aside.
4. Push the onion and garlic to one side of the skillet, then pour the beaten eggs into the other side. Scramble the eggs until cooked through, then mix with the onion and garlic.
5. Add grated cauliflower and thawed peas and carrots to the skillet. Cook, stirring frequently, until the cauliflower is tender, about 5-6 minutes.
6. Stir in cooked shrimp and soy sauce, and cook for an additional 2-3 minutes, until everything is heated through.
7. Season with salt and pepper to taste.
8. Garnish with chopped green onions before serving.

Nutritional Values (Approximate): Calories: 200-250 kcal per serving | Protein: 20-25 grams | Fat: 6-8 grams | Carbohydrates: 15-20 grams | Fiber: 5-7 grams | Sugars: 5-8 grams

Baked Chicken Breast with Quinoa Salad:

Prep Time: 15 minutes   **Cook Time:** 25 minutes   **Servings:** 4

Ingredients:

- 4 boneless, skinless chicken breasts
- 2 tablespoons olive oil
- 1 teaspoon garlic powder
- 1 teaspoon paprika
- Salt and pepper to taste
- 1 cup quinoa, cooked
- 1 cup cherry tomatoes, halved
- 1 cucumber, diced
- 1/4 cup red onion, finely chopped
- 1/4 cup fresh parsley, chopped
- 2 tablespoons lemon juice
- 2 tablespoons extra virgin olive oil
- Salt and pepper to taste

Instructions:

1. Preheat your oven to 400°F (200°C). Line a baking sheet with parchment paper.
2. Place chicken breasts on the prepared baking sheet. Drizzle with olive oil and season with garlic powder, paprika, salt, and pepper.
3. Bake in the preheated oven for 20-25 minutes, or until the chicken is cooked through and no longer pink in the center.
4. While the chicken is baking, prepare the quinoa salad. In a large bowl, combine cooked quinoa, cherry tomatoes, cucumber, red onion, and parsley.
5. In a small bowl, whisk together lemon juice, extra virgin olive oil, salt, and pepper. Pour over the quinoa salad and toss to coat.
6. Once the chicken is cooked, serve it hot with a side of quinoa salad.

Nutritional Values (Approximate): Calories: 300-350 kcal per serving (chicken only) | Protein: 25-30 grams | Fat: 10-12 grams | Carbohydrates: 20-25 grams | Fiber: 3-5 grams | Sugars: 2-4 grams

Prep Time: 20 minutes   **Cook Time:** 20 minutes   **Servings:** 4

Ingredients:

- 1 pound ground turkey
- 1/4 cup breadcrumbs (or almond meal for gluten-free)
- 1/4 cup grated Parmesan cheese
- 1 egg
- 2 cloves garlic, minced
- 2 tablespoons fresh parsley, chopped
- 1 teaspoon dried oregano
- Salt and pepper to taste
- 2 tablespoons olive oil

Ingredients:

- 4 medium zucchini, spiralized
- 2 tablespoons olive oil
- 2 cloves garlic, minced
- Salt and pepper to taste
- Grated Parmesan cheese (optional)

Instructions:

1. Preheat your oven to 400°F (200°C). Line a baking sheet with parchment paper.
2. In a large bowl, combine ground turkey, breadcrumbs, grated Parmesan cheese, egg, minced garlic, chopped parsley, dried oregano, salt, and pepper. Mix until well combined.
3. Shape the mixture into meatballs, about 1-2 inches in diameter.
4. Heat olive oil in a large skillet over medium heat. Add the meatballs and cook until browned on all sides, about 5-7 minutes.
5. Transfer the browned meatballs to the prepared baking sheet and bake in the preheated oven for 12-15 minutes, or until cooked through.

Instructions:

1. While the meatballs are baking, heat olive oil in a large skillet over medium heat. Add minced garlic and cook until fragrant, about 1 minute.

2. Add spiralized zucchini noodles to the skillet and sauté for 3-5 minutes, or until tender.

3. Season with salt and pepper to taste.

4. Serve the turkey meatballs hot over the zucchini noodles.

5. Optional: Garnish with grated Parmesan cheese before serving.

Nutritional Values (Approximate): Calories: 300-350 kcal per serving | Protein: 20-25 grams | Fat: 15-20 grams | Carbohydrates: 15-20 grams | Fiber: 3-5 grams | Sugars: 2-4 grams

Stir-Fried Tofu with Broccoli and Cashews:

Prep Time: 15 minutes   **Cook Time:** 15 minutes   **Servings:** 4

Ingredients:

- 14 oz (400g) extra firm tofu, pressed and cubed
- 2 tablespoons soy sauce
- 1 tablespoon hoisin sauce
- 1 tablespoon sesame oil
- 2 tablespoons vegetable oil
- 3 cloves garlic, minced
- 1 teaspoon ginger, minced
- 2 cups broccoli florets
- 1/2 cup unsalted cashews
- Salt and pepper to taste
- Cooked rice, for serving

Instructions:

1. In a bowl, toss the cubed tofu with soy sauce and hoisin sauce until evenly coated. Let it marinate for about 10 minutes.

2. Heat sesame oil and vegetable oil in a large skillet or wok over medium-high heat.

3. Add minced garlic and ginger to the skillet and sauté for about 1 minute, until fragrant.

4. Add marinated tofu cubes to the skillet. Stir-fry for 5-7 minutes, until the tofu is golden brown and crispy on the edges.

5. Add broccoli florets and cashews to the skillet. Stir-fry for an additional 3-4 minutes, until the broccoli is tender-crisp.

6. Season with salt and pepper to taste.

7. Serve the stir-fried tofu, broccoli, and cashews hot over cooked rice.

Nutritional Values (Approximate): Calories: 250-300 kcal per serving | Protein: 15-20 grams | Fat: 15-20 grams | Carbohydrates: 15-20 grams | Fiber: 3-5 grams | Sugars: 3-5 grams

Prep Time: 20 minutes   **Cook Time:** 40 minutes   **Servings:** 4

Ingredients:

- 2 large eggplants, sliced into rounds
- 1 cup breadcrumbs (or almond meal for gluten-free)
- 1/2 cup grated Parmesan cheese
- 2 eggs, beaten
- 2 cups marinara sauce
- 1 cup shredded mozzarella cheese
- Salt and pepper to taste
- Fresh basil leaves, for garnish

Ingredients:

- 4 cups mixed salad greens (such as spinach, arugula, and lettuce)
- 1 cup cherry tomatoes, halved
- 1/4 cup red onion, thinly sliced
- 2 tablespoons balsamic vinegar
- 2 tablespoons extra virgin olive oil
- Salt and pepper to taste

Instructions:

1. Preheat your oven to 400°F (200°C). Line a baking sheet with parchment paper.

2. In a shallow dish, combine breadcrumbs and grated Parmesan cheese. Season with salt and pepper.

3. Dip eggplant slices into beaten eggs, then coat with breadcrumb mixture.

4. Place coated eggplant slices on the prepared baking sheet. Bake in the preheated oven for 20-25 minutes, or until golden brown and crispy.

5. Spread a thin layer of marinara sauce in the bottom of a baking dish. Arrange baked eggplant slices in a single layer on top of the sauce.

6. Pour the remaining marinara sauce over the eggplant slices. Sprinkle shredded mozzarella cheese on top.

7. Bake in the oven for an additional 15-20 minutes, or until the cheese is melted and bubbly.

8. Garnish with fresh basil leaves before serving.

Instructions:

1. In a large bowl, combine mixed salad greens, cherry tomatoes, and thinly sliced red onion.

2. In a small bowl, whisk together balsamic vinegar, extra virgin olive oil, salt, and pepper.

3. Drizzle the vinaigrette over the salad and toss to coat evenly.

4. Serve the eggplant Parmesan hot with a side of mixed greens salad.

Nutritional Values (Approximate): Calories: 350-400 kcal per serving (eggplant Parmesan only) | Protein: 15-20 grams | Fat: 15-20 grams | Carbohydrates: 30-35 grams | Fiber: 8-10 grams | Sugars: 8-10 grams

Lentil and Vegetable Soup:

Prep Time: 15 minutes   **Cook Time:** 40 minutes   **Servings:** 6

Ingredients:

- 1 cup green lentils, rinsed and drained
- 1 tablespoon olive oil
- 1 onion, diced
- 2 carrots, diced
- 2 celery stalks, diced
- 2 cloves garlic, minced
- 1 teaspoon ground cumin
- 1 teaspoon ground coriander
- 1/2 teaspoon smoked paprika
- 6 cups vegetable broth
- 1 can (14 oz) diced tomatoes
- 2 cups chopped kale or spinach
- Salt and pepper to taste
- Fresh parsley, chopped (for garnish)

Instructions:

1. In a large pot, heat olive oil over medium heat. Add diced onion, carrots, and celery. Sauté until vegetables are softened, about 5-7 minutes.

2. Add minced garlic, ground cumin, ground coriander, and smoked paprika to the pot. Cook for an additional 1-2 minutes, until fragrant.

3. Stir in green lentils, vegetable broth, and diced tomatoes. Bring the soup to a boil, then reduce heat to low. Simmer for about 25-30 minutes, or until lentils are tender.

4. Stir in chopped kale or spinach and cook for an additional 5 minutes, until wilted.

5. Season with salt and pepper to taste.

6. Ladle the lentil and vegetable soup into bowls. Garnish with chopped fresh parsley before serving.

Nutritional Values (Approximate): Calories: 250-300 kcal per serving | Protein: 12-15 grams | Fat: 4-6 grams | Carbohydrates: 40-45 grams | Fiber: 12-15 grams | Sugars: 8-10 grams

Beef and Vegetable Stir-Fry:

Prep Time: 15 minutes   **Cook Time:** 15 minutes   **Servings:** 4

Ingredients:

- 1 lb (450g) beef steak, thinly sliced
- 2 tablespoons soy sauce
- 1 tablespoon oyster sauce
- 1 tablespoon hoisin sauce
- 1 tablespoon sesame oil
- 2 tablespoons vegetable oil
- 3 cloves garlic, minced
- 1-inch piece ginger, minced
- 1 onion, sliced
- 1 bell pepper, sliced
- 1 cup broccoli florets
- 1 carrot, julienned
- Salt and pepper to taste
- Cooked rice or noodles, for serving

Instructions:

1. In a bowl, mix together soy sauce, oyster sauce, hoisin sauce, and sesame oil. Add sliced beef to the mixture and marinate for 10-15 minutes.
2. Heat vegetable oil in a large skillet or wok over high heat.
3. Add minced garlic and ginger to the skillet and stir-fry for 1 minute until fragrant.
4. Add marinated beef to the skillet and stir-fry for 2-3 minutes until browned.
5. Add sliced onion, bell pepper, broccoli florets, and julienned carrot to the skillet. Stir-fry for an additional 3-4 minutes until vegetables are tender-crisp.
6. Season with salt and pepper to taste.
7. Serve the beef and vegetable stir-fry hot over cooked rice or noodles.

Nutritional Values (Approximate): Calories: 300-350 kcal per serving | Protein: 25-30 grams | Fat: 15-20 grams | Carbohydrates: 15-20 grams | Fiber: 3-5 grams | Sugars: 5-8 grams

Spaghetti Squash with Turkey Bolognese:

Prep Time: 15 minutes   **Cook Time:** 1 hour   **Servings:** 4

Ingredients:

- 1 large spaghetti squash
- 1 lb (450g) lean ground turkey
- 1 onion, diced
- 2 cloves garlic, minced
- 1 bell pepper, diced
- 1 carrot, diced
- 1 can (14 oz) diced tomatoes
- 2 tablespoons tomato paste
- 1 teaspoon dried oregano
- 1 teaspoon dried basil
- Salt and pepper to taste
- Fresh basil leaves, for garnish
- Grated Parmesan cheese (optional)

Instructions:

1. Preheat your oven to 400°F (200°C). Cut the spaghetti squash in half lengthwise and scoop out the seeds.

2. Place the squash halves cut-side down on a baking sheet lined with parchment paper. Bake in the preheated oven for 40-45 minutes, or until the squash is tender and easily pierced with a fork.

3. While the squash is baking, heat olive oil in a large skillet over medium heat. Add diced onion, minced garlic, diced bell pepper, and diced carrot. Sauté for 5-7 minutes until vegetables are softened.

4. Add ground turkey to the skillet and cook until browned, breaking it up with a spoon as it cooks.

5. Stir in diced tomatoes, tomato paste, dried oregano, dried basil, salt, and pepper. Simmer for 15-20 minutes until the sauce is thickened.

6. Once the spaghetti squash is cooked, use a fork to scrape the flesh into strands.

7. Serve the spaghetti squash topped with turkey Bolognese sauce.

8. Garnish with fresh basil leaves and grated Parmesan cheese, if desired.

Nutritional Values (Approximate): Calories: 250-300 kcal per serving | Protein: 20-25 grams | Fat: 10-12 grams | Carbohydrates: 20-25 grams | Fiber: 5-7 grams | Sugars: 8-10 grams

Grilled Portobello Mushrooms with Balsamic Glaze:

Prep Time: 10 minutes   **Cook Time:** 10 minutes   **Servings:** 4

Ingredients:

- 4 large portobello mushrooms
- 2 tablespoons balsamic vinegar
- 2 tablespoons olive oil
- 2 cloves garlic, minced
- Salt and pepper to taste
- Fresh parsley, chopped (for garnish)

Instructions:

1. Preheat your grill to medium-high heat.
2. In a small bowl, whisk together balsamic vinegar, olive oil, minced garlic, salt, and pepper.
3. Clean the portobello mushrooms and remove the stems.
4. Brush both sides of the mushrooms with the balsamic marinade.
5. Place the mushrooms on the preheated grill, gill-side down. Grill for 4-5 minutes per side, until tender and grill marks appear.
6. Once cooked, remove the mushrooms from the grill and place them on a serving platter.
7. Drizzle any remaining balsamic marinade over the grilled mushrooms.
8. Garnish with chopped fresh parsley before serving.

Nutritional Values (Approximate): Calories: 80-100 kcal per serving | Protein: 4-6 grams | Fat: 6-8 grams | Carbohydrates: 6-8 grams | Fiber: 2-3 grams | Sugars: 3-5 grams

CHAPTER FIVE:

OMAD Diet Snacks and Desserts

Almonds:

Prep Time: 2 minutes   **Cook Time:** 0 minutes   **Servings:** 1

Ingredients:

- 1/4 cup almonds

Instructions:

1. Simply measure out the almonds.

2. Optionally, you can soak the almonds in water overnight for enhanced digestibility and nutrient absorption.

3. Enjoy as a quick and nutritious snack!

Nutritional Values (Approximate): Calories: 160 kcal | Protein: 6 grams | Fat: 14 grams | Carbohydrates: 6 grams | Fiber: 3 grams | Sugars: 1 gram

Baby Carrots with Hummus:

Prep Time: 5 minutes **Cook Time:** 0 minutes **Servings:** 1

Ingredients:

- 1/2 cup baby carrots
- 2 tablespoons hummus

Instructions:

1. Rinse the baby carrots under cold water and pat them dry.

2. Arrange the baby carrots on a plate or in a small bowl.

3. Serve alongside the hummus for dipping.

4. Enjoy as a healthy and crunchy snack!

Nutritional Values (Approximate): Calories: 70 kcal | Protein: 2 grams | Fat: 3 grams | Carbohydrates: 10 grams | Fiber: 3 grams | Sugars: 4 grams

Greek Yogurt with Honey:

Prep Time: 2 minutes   **Cook Time:** 0 minutes   **Servings:** 1

Ingredients:

- 1/2 cup Greek yogurt
- 1 tablespoon honey

Instructions:

1. Spoon the Greek yogurt into a serving bowl.
2. Drizzle the honey over the Greek yogurt.
3. Stir gently to combine.
4. Enjoy as a creamy and satisfying dessert or snack!

Nutritional Values (Approximate): Calories: 150 kcal

| Protein: 12 grams | Fat: 0 grams | Carbohydrates: 22 grams | Fiber: 0 grams | Sugars: 20 grams

Sliced Cucumbers with Cottage Cheese:

Prep Time: 5 minutes   **Cook Time:** 0 minutes   **Servings:** 1

Ingredients:

- 1/2 cucumber, sliced

- 1/4 cup cottage cheese

Instructions:

1. Wash the cucumber and slice it into rounds or sticks.

2. Arrange the cucumber slices on a plate.

3. Serve alongside the cottage cheese.

4. Enjoy this refreshing and protein-packed snack!

Nutritional Values (Approximate): Calories: 90 kcal | Protein: 11 grams | Fat: 1 gram | Carbohydrates: 9 grams | Fiber: 2 grams | Sugars: 5 grams

Apple Slices with Almond Butter:

Prep Time: 5 minutes   **Cook Time:** 0 minutes   **Servings:** 1

Ingredients:

- 1 medium apple
- 2 tablespoons almond butter

Instructions:

1. Wash the apple and slice it into thin wedges.
2. Arrange the apple slices on a plate.
3. Spoon the almond butter into a small bowl for dipping.
4. Dip the apple slices into the almond butter.
5. Enjoy this delicious and satisfying snack!

Nutritional Values (Approximate): Calories: 250 kcal | Protein: 5 grams | Fat: 14 grams | Carbohydrates: 28 grams | Fiber: 6 grams | Sugars: 18 grams

Celery Sticks with Peanut Butter:

Prep Time: 5 minutes   **Cook Time:** 0 minutes   **Servings:** 1

Ingredients:

- 2 stalks of celery
- 2 tablespoons peanut butter

Instructions:

1. Wash the celery stalks and cut them into manageable sticks.
2. Spread peanut butter onto each celery stick.
3. Arrange the celery sticks on a plate.
4. Enjoy this crunchy and satisfying snack!

Nutritional Values (Approximate): Calories: 200 kcal | Protein: 7 grams | Fat: 16 grams | Carbohydrates: 8 grams | Fiber: 4 grams | Sugars: 3 grams

Hard-Boiled Eggs:

Prep Time: 5 minutes   **Cook Time:** 10 minutes   **Servings:** 1

Ingredients:

- 2 large eggs

Instructions:

1. Place the eggs in a saucepan and cover them with cold water.
2. Bring the water to a boil over medium-high heat.
3. Once boiling, cover the saucepan and remove it from the heat.
4. Let the eggs sit in the hot water for 10 minutes.
5. After 10 minutes, transfer the eggs to a bowl of ice water to cool.
6. Once cooled, peel the eggs and enjoy as a protein-rich snack!

Nutritional Values (Approximate): Calories: 140 kcal | Protein: 12 grams | Fat: 10 grams | Carbohydrates: 1 gram | Fiber: 0 grams | Sugars: 0 grams

Cherry Tomatoes with Mozzarella Cheese:

Prep Time: 5 minutes   **Cook Time:** 0 minutes   **Servings:** 1

Ingredients:

- 1/2 cup cherry tomatoes
- 1/4 cup fresh mozzarella cheese balls
- Fresh basil leaves for garnish (optional)
- Balsamic glaze for drizzling (optional)

Instructions:

1. Rinse the cherry tomatoes and pat them dry with a paper towel.
2. Arrange the cherry tomatoes and mozzarella cheese balls on a serving plate.
3. Garnish with fresh basil leaves if desired.
4. Drizzle with balsamic glaze for added flavor if desired.
5. Enjoy this colorful and flavorful snack!

Nutritional Values (Approximate): Calories: 120 kcal | Protein: 6 grams | Fat: 8 grams | Carbohydrates: 5 grams | Fiber: 1 gram | Sugars: 3 grams

Edamame Beans:

Prep Time: 5 minutes   **Cook Time:** 5 minutes   **Servings:** 1

Ingredients:

- 1 cup frozen edamame beans (in pods)
- Sea salt for sprinkling (optional)

Instructions:

1. Bring a pot of water to a boil over high heat.
2. Add the frozen edamame beans to the boiling water.
3. Cook for 4-5 minutes, or until the beans are tender.
4. Drain the beans and transfer them to a serving bowl.
5. Sprinkle with sea salt if desired.
6. Enjoy this protein-packed and nutritious snack!

Nutritional Values (Approximate): Calories: 120 kcal | Protein: 11 grams | Fat: 4 grams | Carbohydrates: 10 grams | Fiber: 6 grams | Sugars: 2 grams

Whole Grain Crackers with Avocado:

Prep Time: 5 minutes   **Cook Time:** 0 minutes   **Servings:** 1

Ingredients:

- 4 whole grain crackers
- 1/2 ripe avocado
- Pinch of sea salt
- Optional toppings: sliced radishes, cherry tomatoes, or sprouts

Instructions:

1. Slice the avocado in half and remove the pit.
2. Scoop out the avocado flesh and mash it with a fork in a small bowl.
3. Spread the mashed avocado onto each whole grain cracker.

4. Sprinkle a pinch of sea salt over the avocado.

5. Top with sliced radishes, cherry tomatoes, or sprouts if desired.

6. Enjoy this satisfying and nutrient-rich snack!

Nutritional Values (Approximate): Calories: 200 kcal | Protein: 4 grams | Fat: 12 grams | Carbohydrates: 20 grams | Fiber: 8 grams | Sugars: 1 gram

Fresh Fruit Salad:

Prep Time: 10 minutes   **Servings:** 4

Ingredients:

- 2 cups mixed fresh fruits (such as strawberries, pineapple, grapes, kiwi, oranges, and mango)
- 2 tablespoons fresh mint leaves, chopped
- 1 tablespoon honey
- 1 tablespoon lemon juice

Instructions:

1. Wash and prepare the fruits as needed. Cut larger fruits into bite-sized pieces.

2. In a large bowl, combine the mixed fresh fruits and chopped mint leaves.

3. Drizzle honey and lemon juice over the fruit mixture.

4. Gently toss the fruits until evenly coated with the honey and lemon juice.

5. Serve immediately or refrigerate until ready to serve.

Nutritional Values (Approximate): Calories: 80-100 kcal | Protein: 1-2 grams | Fat: 0 grams | Carbohydrates: 20-25 grams | Fiber: 2-4 grams | Sugars: 15-20 grams

Greek Yogurt Parfait with Granola and Berries:

Prep Time: 5 minutes   **Servings:** 2

Ingredients:

- 1 cup Greek yogurt
- 1/2 cup granola
- 1/2 cup mixed berries (such as strawberries, blueberries, raspberries)
- 2 tablespoons honey (optional)

Instructions:

1. In two serving glasses or bowls, layer the Greek yogurt, granola, and mixed berries.
2. Repeat the layers until the glasses or bowls are filled, ending with a layer of mixed berries on top.
3. Drizzle honey over the top layer, if desired.
4. Serve immediately, or refrigerate until ready to serve.

Nutritional Values (Approximate): Calories: 250-300 kcal | Protein: 10-12 grams | Fat: 5-7 grams | Carbohydrates: 40-45 grams | Fiber: 4-6 grams | Sugars: 25-30 grams

Chia Seed Pudding with Coconut Milk and Mango:

Prep Time: 5 minutes (+overnight soaking)   **Servings:** 2

Ingredients:

- 1/4 cup chia seeds
- 1 cup coconut milk
- 1 tablespoon honey or maple syrup (optional)
- 1 ripe mango, diced

Instructions:

1. In a mixing bowl, combine chia seeds and coconut milk. If desired, add honey or maple syrup for sweetness.
2. Stir well to combine, ensuring that the chia seeds are evenly distributed.
3. Cover the bowl and refrigerate overnight, or for at least 4 hours, to allow the chia seeds to thicken and absorb the liquid.

4. Before serving, stir the pudding to ensure the consistency is smooth.

5. Divide the chia seed pudding into serving bowls or glasses.

6. Top with diced mango.

7. Serve chilled.

Nutritional Values (Approximate): Calories: 200-250 kcal | Protein: 4-6 grams | Fat: 10-12 grams | Carbohydrates: 25-30 grams | Fiber: 8-10 grams | Sugars: 15-20 grams

Baked Apples with Cinnamon and a Dollop of Greek Yogurt:

Prep Time: 10 minutes   **Cook Time:** 30 minutes   **Servings:** 2

Ingredients:

- 2 apples (such as Granny Smith or Honeycrisp)
- 1 teaspoon cinnamon
- 1 tablespoon honey (optional)
- 2 tablespoons Greek yogurt

Instructions:

1. Preheat the oven to 375°F (190°C).
2. Core the apples and cut them in half horizontally.
3. Place the apple halves, cut side up, on a baking dish.
4. Sprinkle cinnamon over the apple halves. If desired, drizzle honey over the top for extra sweetness.
5. Bake in the preheated oven for about 25-30 minutes, or until the apples are tender.
6. Remove the baked apples from the oven and let them cool slightly.
7. Serve the baked apples warm with a dollop of Greek yogurt on top.
8. Optionally, you can sprinkle additional cinnamon over the yogurt before serving.

Nutritional Values (Approximate): Calories: 150-200 kcal | Protein: 2-4 grams | Fat: 0-2 grams | Carbohydrates: 35-40 grams | Fiber: 6-8 grams | Sugars: 25-30 grams

Frozen Banana Slices Dipped in Dark Chocolate:

Prep Time: 15 minutes (+freezing time)   **Servings:** 4

Ingredients:

- 2 ripe bananas
- 4 ounces dark chocolate, chopped
- 1 tablespoon coconut oil (optional)
- Toppings of your choice (e.g., chopped nuts, shredded coconut, sprinkles)

Instructions:

1. Peel the bananas and cut them into thick slices.
2. Place the banana slices on a parchment-lined baking sheet and freeze for at least 1 hour, or until firm.
3. In a microwave-safe bowl, combine the chopped dark chocolate and coconut oil (if using). Microwave in 30-second intervals, stirring in between, until the chocolate is melted and smooth.
4. Dip each frozen banana slice into the melted chocolate, using a fork to coat it completely. Allow any excess chocolate to drip off.
5. Place the chocolate-covered banana slices back onto the parchment-lined baking sheet.
6. Immediately sprinkle your desired toppings over the chocolate before it sets.
7. Return the baking sheet to the freezer and freeze until the chocolate is firm, about 30 minutes.
8. Once the chocolate is set, transfer the frozen banana slices to an airtight container and store in the freezer until ready to serve.

Nutritional Values (Approximate): Calories: 150-200 kcal | Protein: 2-4 grams | Fat: 8-10 grams | Carbohydrates: 20-25 grams | Fiber: 3-5 grams | Sugars: 12-15 grams

Mixed Berry Sorbet Made with Frozen Berries and a Splash of Lemon Juice:

Prep Time: 5 minutes (+freezing time)   **Servings:** 2

Ingredients:

- 2 cups mixed frozen berries (such as strawberries, blueberries, raspberries)
- 1 tablespoon lemon juice
- 1-2 tablespoons honey or maple syrup (optional)

Instructions:

1. Place the frozen berries, lemon juice, and honey or maple syrup (if using) in a food processor or blender.
2. Blend the mixture until smooth and creamy. You may need to stop and scrape down the sides of the blender occasionally.
3. Taste the sorbet mixture and adjust the sweetness, if desired, by adding more honey or maple syrup.
4. Once the sorbet reaches your desired consistency and taste, transfer it to a freezer-safe container.
5. Cover the container and freeze the sorbet for at least 2-3 hours, or until firm.
6. Before serving, let the sorbet sit at room temperature for a few minutes to soften slightly.
7. Scoop the mixed berry sorbet into bowls or serving glasses and enjoy!

Nutritional Values (Approximate): Calories: 80-100 kcal | Protein: 1-2 grams | Fat: 0-1 grams | Carbohydrates: 20-25 grams | Fiber: 5-7 grams | Sugars: 10-15 grams

Coconut Milk Panna Cotta with Raspberry Coulis:

Prep Time: 10 minutes (+chilling time)   **Cook Time:** 10 minutes

Servings: 4

Ingredients for Panna Cotta:

- 1 can (13.5 oz) coconut milk
- 2 tablespoons honey or maple syrup
- 1 teaspoon vanilla extract
- 1 packet (about 2 1/4 teaspoons) unflavored gelatin
- 2 tablespoons cold water

Ingredients for Raspberry Coulis:

- 1 cup fresh or frozen raspberries
- 2 tablespoons honey or maple syrup
- 1 tablespoon lemon juice

Instructions for Panna Cotta:

1. In a small bowl, sprinkle the gelatin over cold water and let it sit for about 5 minutes to bloom.
2. In a saucepan, heat the coconut milk and honey (or maple syrup) over medium heat until just simmering. Remove from heat and stir in the vanilla extract.
3. Add the bloomed gelatin to the warm coconut milk mixture and stir until completely dissolved.
4. Divide the mixture evenly among four ramekins or serving glasses.
5. Refrigerate for at least 4 hours, or until set.

Instructions for Raspberry Coulis:

1. In a small saucepan, combine the raspberries, honey (or maple syrup), and lemon juice.
2. Cook over medium heat, stirring occasionally, until the raspberries break down and the mixture thickens slightly, about 5-7 minutes.
3. Remove from heat and let cool slightly.
4. Transfer the raspberry mixture to a blender or food processor and blend until smooth.
5. Strain the coulis through a fine-mesh sieve to remove the seeds, if desired.

6. Allow the coulis to cool completely before serving.

To Serve:

1. Once the panna cotta is set, carefully run a knife around the edge of each ramekin or glass to loosen it.

2. Dip the bottom of each ramekin or glass in hot water for a few seconds to help release the panna cotta.

3. Invert each ramekin or glass onto a serving plate to unmold the panna cotta.

4. Drizzle the raspberry coulis over the top of each panna cotta just before serving.

5. Garnish with fresh raspberries or mint leaves, if desired.

6. Serve and enjoy!

Nutritional Values (Approximate): Calories: 250-300 kcal | Protein: 3-5 grams | Fat: 20-25 grams | Carbohydrates: 20-25 grams | Fiber: 3-5 grams | Sugars: 15-20 grams

Chocolate Avocado Mousse:

Prep Time: 10 minutes (+chilling time)   **Servings:** 2-4

Ingredients:

- 2 ripe avocados
- 1/4 cup cocoa powder
- 1/4 cup honey or maple syrup
- 1 teaspoon vanilla extract
- Pinch of salt
- Optional toppings: shaved chocolate, berries, whipped cream

Instructions:

1. Cut the avocados in half and remove the pits. Scoop the flesh into a blender or food processor.

2. Add cocoa powder, honey (or maple syrup), vanilla extract, and a pinch of salt to the blender or food processor.

3. Blend until smooth and creamy, scraping down the sides as needed to ensure everything is well incorporated.

4. Taste and adjust sweetness if necessary by adding more honey or maple syrup.

5. Transfer the chocolate avocado mixture to serving bowls or glasses.

6. Cover and refrigerate for at least 1-2 hours, or until chilled and set.

7. Before serving, garnish with toppings of your choice, such as shaved chocolate, berries, or whipped cream.

8. Serve and enjoy!

Nutritional Values (Approximate): Calories: 200-250 kcal | Protein: 3-5 grams | Fat: 15-20 grams | Carbohydrates: 25-30 grams | Fiber: 7-10 grams | Sugars: 15-20 grams

Baked Peaches with a Sprinkle of Cinnamon and a Drizzle of Honey:

Prep Time: 10 minutes   **Cook Time:** 20 minutes   Cook Time: 4

Ingredients:

- 4 ripe peaches
- 1 teaspoon ground cinnamon
- 2 tablespoons honey
- Optional: vanilla ice cream or Greek yogurt for serving

Instructions:

1. Preheat your oven to 375°F (190°C) and line a baking sheet with parchment paper.

2. Cut the peaches in half and remove the pits. Place the peach halves cut-side up on the prepared baking sheet.

3. Sprinkle each peach half with ground cinnamon.

4. Drizzle honey over the top of each peach half.

5. Bake in the preheated oven for about 15-20 minutes, or until the peaches are soft and juicy.

6. Remove from the oven and let cool slightly before serving.

7. Serve the baked peaches warm with a scoop of vanilla ice cream or a dollop of Greek yogurt, if desired.

Nutritional Values (Approximate): Calories: 80-100 kcal | Protein: 1-2 grams | Fat: 0-1 grams | Carbohydrates: 20-25 grams | Fiber: 2-3 grams | Sugars: 15-20 grams

Mango Coconut Ice Pops:

Prep Time: 10 minutes (+freezing time)   **Servings:** 6

Ingredients:

- 2 ripe mangoes, peeled and diced
- 1 cup coconut milk
- 2 tablespoons honey or maple syrup (optional)
- 1 teaspoon vanilla extract
- 1/4 cup shredded coconut (optional)

Instructions:

1. Place the diced mangoes, coconut milk, honey (or maple syrup), and vanilla extract in a blender.
2. Blend until smooth and creamy.
3. If desired, stir in shredded coconut for added texture.
4. Pour the mango coconut mixture into ice pop molds, leaving a little space at the top for expansion.
5. Insert ice pop sticks into the molds.
6. Place the molds in the freezer and freeze for at least 4-6 hours, or until completely frozen.
7. Once frozen, remove the ice pops from the molds by running them under warm water for a few seconds.
8. Serve immediately and enjoy!

Nutritional Values (Approximate): Calories: 100-120 kcal | Protein: 1-2 grams | Fat: 6-8 grams | Carbohydrates: 15-20 grams | Fiber: 2-3 grams | Sugars: 10-15 grams

CHAPTER SIX:

Tips for Success on the OMAD Diet

1. **Understand the OMAD Concept**: Before starting the OMAD diet, it's crucial to fully grasp the concept. OMAD involves consuming all your daily calories, nutrients, and hydration within a single meal window, typically lasting around one hour.

2. **Consult with a Healthcare Professional**: As with any major dietary change, it's essential to consult with a healthcare professional, especially if you have any underlying health conditions or concerns. They can provide personalized advice and ensure the OMAD approach is suitable for you.

3. **Choose Nutrient-Dense Foods**: Since you're eating only one meal a day, make every bite count by choosing nutrient-dense foods. Focus on incorporating lean proteins, healthy fats, whole grains, fruits, vegetables, and legumes to ensure you're meeting your nutritional needs.

4. **Hydration is Key**: Staying hydrated is crucial on the OMAD diet. While you're fasting throughout the day, make sure to drink plenty of water to maintain hydration levels. Herbal teas, black coffee, and sparkling water are also acceptable options during the fasting period.

5. **Plan Your Meals Wisely**: Planning is essential when following the OMAD diet. Take the time to plan your meal in advance, ensuring it's balanced and provides all the essential nutrients your body needs. Consider meal prepping to make it easier to stick to your eating window.

6. **Listen to Your Body**: Pay attention to your body's hunger and fullness cues. Since you're eating only one meal a day, it's crucial to tune in to your body's signals to avoid overeating or undereating during your meal window.

7. **Slow Down and Enjoy Your Meal**: Since you're eating only one meal, take the time to savor each bite and fully enjoy your food. Eating mindfully can help you feel more satisfied and prevent the urge to overeat.

8. **Consider Macronutrient Balance**: While there are no strict rules about macronutrient ratios on the OMAD diet, many people find success by including a balance of protein, healthy fats, and carbohydrates in their meals. Experiment with different ratios to find what works best for you.

9. **Stay Flexible**: While OMAD is typically practiced daily, it's essential to listen to your body and be flexible with your approach. Some days you may need to adjust your eating window or include a snack if you're feeling particularly hungry or fatigued.

10. **Monitor Your Progress**: Keep track of your progress on the OMAD diet, including how you feel physically, mentally, and any changes in weight or body composition. Adjust your approach as needed based on your individual goals and experiences.

AMOUNT OF EXERCISE

The amount of exercise recommended during the OMAD (One Meal A Day) diet can vary depending on individual goals, fitness levels, and preferences. However, here are some general guidelines to consider:

1. **Moderate Aerobic Exercise**: Aim for at least 150 minutes of moderate-intensity aerobic exercise per week, such as brisk walking, cycling, swimming, or dancing. This can be divided into 30-minute sessions on most days of the week. Moderate-intensity exercise should elevate your heart rate and breathing, but still allow you to carry on a conversation.

2. **Strength Training**: Include strength training exercises at least two days per week. Focus on major muscle groups, including the chest, back, arms, shoulders, legs, and core. Use resistance bands, free weights, machines, or bodyweight exercises like squats, lunges, push-ups, and planks. Aim for 8-12 repetitions of each exercise, performing 2-3 sets.

3. **High-Intensity Interval Training (HIIT)**: Incorporate HIIT workouts 1-2 times per week for added calorie burn and cardiovascular benefits. HIIT involves alternating between short bursts of high-intensity exercise (e.g., sprinting, jumping jacks, burpees) and periods of rest or low-intensity exercise. A typical HIIT session may last 20-30 minutes, including warm-up and cool-down.

4. **Flexibility and Mobility**: Don't forget to include flexibility and mobility exercises in your routine to improve joint range of motion, prevent injury, and promote relaxation. Incorporate stretching, yoga, or Pilates exercises at least 2-3 times per week, focusing on major muscle groups and areas of tightness or discomfort.

5. **Listen to Your Body**: Pay attention to your body's signals and adjust the intensity, duration, and frequency of exercise based on how you feel. Some days you may have more energy and motivation for longer or more intense workouts, while other days you may need to take it easy and focus on gentle movement or restorative activities.

6. **Be Consistent and Gradual**: Consistency is key when it comes to exercise, especially during the OMAD diet. Aim to establish a regular exercise routine that you can realistically stick to over the long term. Start gradually, especially if you're new to exercise or returning after a period of inactivity, and gradually increase the intensity and duration as your fitness improves.

7. **Stay Hydrated and Fueled**: Since you're following the OMAD diet, it's important to stay hydrated and properly fueled for your workouts. Drink plenty of water throughout the day, especially before and after exercise, to maintain hydration levels. Additionally,

consider timing your meal to provide adequate energy and nutrients for optimal performance during your workouts.

BENEFITS OF EXERCISE

1. **Enhanced Fat Loss**: Exercise, particularly cardiovascular and strength training exercises, can enhance fat loss when combined with the OMAD diet. By creating a calorie deficit through exercise and consuming your meal within a restricted time frame, your body is more likely to tap into stored fat for energy during the fasting period.

2. **Preservation of Lean Muscle Mass**: Regular exercise, especially resistance training, helps preserve lean muscle mass while on the OMAD diet. This is important for maintaining metabolic rate and preventing muscle loss, which can occur during periods of calorie restriction or fasting.

3. **Improved Metabolic Health**: Exercise has been shown to improve insulin sensitivity, glucose metabolism, and lipid profiles, all of which contribute to better metabolic health. When combined with the OMAD diet, exercise can enhance these metabolic benefits, potentially reducing the risk of insulin resistance, type 2 diabetes, and cardiovascular disease.

4. **Increased Energy Levels**: Contrary to common misconceptions, exercise can actually increase energy levels, even when following a fasting protocol like OMAD. Regular physical activity stimulates the release of endorphins, improves circulation, and boosts overall energy levels, helping you feel more energized throughout the day.

5. **Enhanced Mood and Mental Well-being**: Exercise is known to have mood-boosting effects due to the release of neurotransmitters like endorphins and serotonin. Engaging in regular physical activity while on the OMAD diet can help alleviate stress, anxiety, and depression, promoting overall mental well-being.

6. **Better Appetite Regulation**: Exercise can help regulate appetite and hunger hormones, such as ghrelin and leptin, which may be beneficial when practicing OMAD. By engaging in physical activity, you may experience improved appetite control, reduced cravings, and better adherence to your eating window.

7. **Increased Fat Oxidation**: Exercise enhances the body's ability to oxidize fat for fuel, a process known as fat oxidation. When combined with the OMAD diet, exercise can optimize fat-burning mechanisms, leading to greater fat loss and improved body composition over time.

8. **Long-Term Weight Maintenance**: Incorporating exercise into your routine while following the OMAD diet can support long-term weight maintenance and overall health. Regular physical activity helps sustain weight loss, prevents weight regain, and promotes a healthy body composition, contributing to sustainable lifestyle changes.

It's important to note that the benefits of exercise during the OMAD diet may vary depending on individual factors such as fitness level, exercise intensity, duration, and frequency. Always listen to your body, consult with a healthcare professional before starting any new exercise program, and adjust your routine based on your personal goals and preferences.

RAPID FAT LOSS EXERCISE

When aiming for rapid fat loss through exercise, it's important to focus on workouts that maximize calorie burn, increase metabolic rate, and promote fat oxidation. Here are some effective types of exercise for rapid fat loss:

1. **High-Intensity Interval Training (HIIT)**: HIIT workouts involve short bursts of intense exercise followed by brief periods of rest or low-intensity recovery. This type of training is highly effective for burning calories both during and after the workout, known as the "afterburn" effect or excess post-exercise oxygen consumption (EPOC). HIIT can be performed with various exercises such as sprints, jumping jacks, burpees, or cycling.

2. **Resistance Training**: Incorporating strength training exercises into your routine can help build lean muscle mass, which in turn increases metabolic rate and promotes fat loss. Focus on compound exercises that target multiple muscle groups simultaneously, such as squats, deadlifts, lunges, bench presses, and rows. Aim for higher repetitions and shorter rest periods to keep the intensity high and maximize calorie burn.

3. **Cardiovascular Exercise**: While HIIT is a form of cardiovascular exercise, steady-state cardio workouts can also be beneficial for burning calories and promoting fat loss, especially when performed at moderate to high intensity. Activities like running, cycling, swimming, or using cardio machines like the treadmill or elliptical can help increase calorie expenditure and improve cardiovascular health.

4. **Circuit Training**: Circuit training combines strength training and cardiovascular exercise into a single, high-intensity workout. Perform a series of resistance exercises back-to-back with minimal rest in between, incorporating bodyweight exercises, free weights, or resistance bands. This type of workout maximizes calorie burn, builds strength, and improves cardiovascular fitness simultaneously.

5. **Interval Running**: Incorporate interval running sessions into your routine to increase calorie burn and improve cardiovascular fitness. Alternate between periods of high-intensity running or sprinting and recovery periods of walking or jogging. Interval running can be performed outdoors or on a treadmill and can be customized to your fitness level and goals.

6. **Functional Training**: Functional training focuses on movements that mimic real-life activities and improve overall strength, stability, and mobility. Incorporate exercises like

kettlebell swings, battle ropes, medicine ball slams, and plyometric movements to engage multiple muscle groups and burn more calories.

7. **Group Fitness Classes**: Group fitness classes such as spinning, boot camp, or circuit training classes can provide motivation, accountability, and a structured workout environment conducive to fat loss. These classes often incorporate a combination of cardio and strength exercises designed to maximize calorie burn and improve overall fitness.

8. **Consistency and Progression**: Consistency is key when it comes to rapid fat loss through exercise. Aim to exercise most days of the week, gradually increasing the intensity, duration, and frequency of your workouts as your fitness level improves. Incorporate variety into your routine to prevent plateaus and keep your body challenged.

Remember that while exercise is an important component of fat loss, it should be combined with a healthy diet, adequate hydration, and sufficient rest and recovery for optimal results. Additionally, it's essential to listen to your body, prioritize safety, and consult with a healthcare professional before starting any new exercise program, especially if you have any underlying health conditions or concerns.

WEIGHING FREQUENTLY

Weighing yourself frequently can be a useful tool for tracking progress and staying accountable on your weight loss journey, including during the OMAD (One Meal A Day) diet. However, it's essential to approach frequent weighing with a balanced mindset and understand its potential benefits and limitations. Here are some considerations:

Benefits of Weighing Frequently:

1. **Track Progress**: Regular weigh-ins allow you to monitor changes in your weight over time, providing valuable feedback on the effectiveness of your diet and exercise regimen. This can help you stay motivated and make adjustments as needed to reach your goals.

2. **Identify Patterns**: By weighing yourself frequently, you may be able to identify patterns or trends in your weight fluctuations, such as fluctuations related to menstrual cycles, hydration levels, or dietary choices. This insight can help you make informed decisions about your lifestyle and behaviors.

3. **Stay Accountable**: Knowing that you'll be weighing yourself regularly can help keep you accountable to your weight loss goals. It may serve as a reminder to make healthier choices and stick to your plan, knowing that you'll have to face the scale regularly.

4. **Prevent Plateaus**: Monitoring your weight frequently can help you identify and address plateaus more quickly. If you notice your weight stagnating, you can adjust your diet, exercise, or other lifestyle factors to kickstart progress again.

Limitations and Considerations:

1. **Day-to-Day Fluctuations**: It's important to recognize that weight can fluctuate from day to day due to factors like water retention, bowel movements, and food intake. These fluctuations are normal and may not accurately reflect changes in body fat.

2. **Focus on Trends**: Instead of fixating on daily fluctuations, focus on long-term trends in your weight. Look for overall patterns of weight loss or maintenance over the course of several weeks or months, rather than getting discouraged by minor fluctuations.

3. **Emotional Impact**: For some individuals, frequent weighing can lead to anxiety, frustration, or obsessive behavior around food and weight. If weighing yourself frequently negatively affects your mental well-being or leads to disordered eating patterns, it may be best to limit or avoid frequent weigh-ins.

4. **Use Other Measures of Progress**: While weight is one measure of progress, it's not the only indicator of health and fitness. Consider incorporating other measures such as body measurements, progress photos, fitness assessments, and how you feel physically and mentally.

5. **Choose the Right Time**: For more consistent results, weigh yourself at the same time of day under similar conditions, such as in the morning after using the bathroom and before eating or drinking.

CHAPTER SEVEN:

LIFESTYLE

HIDDEN FACTORS

Hidden factors refer to underlying or lesser-known influences that can affect various aspects of health and well-being, including weight loss, metabolism, and overall health. These factors may not always be immediately obvious or apparent but can play a significant role in shaping individual health outcomes. Here are some common hidden factors that may impact weight loss and overall health:

1. **Genetic Predispositions**: Genetic factors can influence metabolism, appetite regulation, fat storage, and other physiological processes related to weight management. Certain genetic variations may make individuals more prone to weight gain or obesity and may also affect how they respond to different dietary and lifestyle interventions.

2. **Hormonal Imbalances**: Hormones play a crucial role in regulating metabolism, appetite, energy balance, and fat storage. Imbalances in hormones such as insulin, cortisol, thyroid hormones, estrogen, testosterone, and leptin can disrupt these processes and contribute to weight gain or difficulty losing weight.

3. **Stress and Emotional Health**: Chronic stress, anxiety, depression, and other emotional factors can impact eating behaviors, food choices, metabolism, and overall health. Stress hormones like cortisol can promote abdominal fat accumulation and increase appetite, while emotional eating may lead to overeating and weight gain.

4. **Sleep Quality and Sleep Disorders**: Poor sleep quality, insufficient sleep, or sleep disorders such as sleep apnea can disrupt hormone regulation, appetite control, and metabolic function. Sleep deprivation can increase hunger hormones like ghrelin and decrease satiety hormones like leptin, leading to overeating and weight gain.

5. **Nutritional Deficiencies**: Deficiencies in essential nutrients such as vitamins, minerals, and omega-3 fatty acids can affect metabolism, energy production, and overall health. Nutrient deficiencies may result from inadequate dietary intake, poor absorption, or increased nutrient requirements due to factors like stress, illness, or certain medications.

6. **Gut Health and Microbiome Composition**: The gut microbiome, consisting of trillions of microorganisms living in the digestive tract, plays a crucial role in digestion, nutrient absorption, metabolism, and immune function. Imbalances in gut bacteria or dysbiosis have been linked to obesity, insulin resistance, inflammation, and other health issues.

7. **Food Sensitivities and Allergies**: Undiagnosed food sensitivities or allergies can trigger immune reactions, inflammation, digestive problems, and other symptoms that may hinder weight loss or contribute to overall health issues. Common culprits include gluten, dairy, soy, eggs, and certain additives or preservatives.

8. **Medication Side Effects**: Some medications, including certain antidepressants, antipsychotics, corticosteroids, and beta-blockers, may have side effects that affect appetite, metabolism, energy levels, or weight regulation. It's essential to be aware of potential medication-related factors that may impact weight management.

9. **Environmental Toxins**: Exposure to environmental toxins such as endocrine-disrupting chemicals (EDCs), heavy metals, pesticides, and air pollutants can interfere with hormone balance, metabolism, and overall health. These toxins may accumulate in the body over time and contribute to weight gain, insulin resistance, and other metabolic disturbances.

10. **Lifestyle Factors**: Sedentary behavior, excessive sitting, lack of physical activity, irregular eating patterns, and poor dietary habits can all influence weight management and overall health. Addressing lifestyle factors such as stress management, sleep hygiene, exercise, and healthy eating habits is essential for long-term weight loss success.

TESTING FOR HIDDEN FACTORS

Testing for hidden factors that may affect weight loss or overall health can be valuable for identifying underlying issues and making informed decisions about your diet, lifestyle, and treatment options. Here are some common tests and assessments that can help uncover hidden factors:

1. **Comprehensive Blood Panel**: A comprehensive blood panel, including tests such as fasting glucose, lipid profile (cholesterol levels), thyroid function tests (TSH, T3, T4), liver function tests (AST, ALT), and markers of inflammation (CRP, ESR), can provide valuable insights into your metabolic health, hormone levels, and overall well-being.

2. **Nutritional Deficiency Testing**: Testing for nutritional deficiencies, such as vitamin D, vitamin B12, iron, magnesium, and omega-3 fatty acids, can identify imbalances that may impact energy levels, metabolism, and overall health. Nutritional deficiencies can occur even in individuals following a seemingly healthy diet.

3. **Food Sensitivity Testing**: Food sensitivity testing can help identify specific foods or ingredients that may be triggering inflammation, digestive issues, or other symptoms that could hinder weight loss or contribute to overall health problems. Common tests include IgG antibody testing or elimination diets followed by food reintroduction.

4. **Gut Health Assessment**: Assessing gut health through tests such as comprehensive stool analysis or gut microbiome testing can provide insights into the balance of beneficial

and harmful bacteria in the digestive system. Imbalances in gut flora have been linked to various health issues, including weight gain, inflammation, and autoimmune conditions.

5. **Hormone Testing**: Hormone imbalances, such as insulin resistance, cortisol dysregulation, or sex hormone imbalances (e.g., estrogen, testosterone), can impact metabolism, appetite regulation, and body composition. Hormone testing, including saliva, blood, or urine tests, can help identify underlying issues that may be contributing to weight loss resistance.

6. **Sleep Assessment**: Poor sleep quality or sleep disorders such as sleep apnea can interfere with weight loss efforts and overall health. A sleep assessment, including sleep quality questionnaires or a polysomnography test (overnight sleep study), can help identify sleep-related issues that may need to be addressed.

7. **Stress Management Assessment**: Chronic stress can disrupt hormone balance, increase inflammation, and contribute to weight gain or difficulty losing weight. Assessing stress levels through questionnaires, cortisol testing (saliva or blood), or heart rate variability (HRV) monitoring can help identify stress-related factors that may be impacting health and well-being.

8. **Medical History and Physical Examination**: A thorough medical history and physical examination by a healthcare professional can provide important clues about underlying health conditions, genetic predispositions, lifestyle factors, and other considerations that may influence weight loss and overall health.

9. **Genetic Testing**: Genetic testing, such as DNA analysis through companies like 23andMe or AncestryDNA, can provide insights into genetic factors that may affect metabolism, nutrient metabolism, appetite regulation, and other aspects of health. However, interpretation of genetic testing results should be done in consultation with a qualified healthcare professional.

10. **Functional Medicine Assessment**: A functional medicine approach involves a comprehensive evaluation of multiple body systems, including lifestyle factors, diet, stress levels, sleep quality, environmental exposures, and genetic predispositions. Functional medicine practitioners use a combination of conventional and alternative testing methods to identify underlying imbalances and develop personalized treatment plans.

BLOOD SUGAR AND INSULIN

Blood Sugar (Glucose):

- Glucose is the primary source of energy for the body's cells, particularly the brain.

- When you eat carbohydrates, they are broken down into glucose, which enters the bloodstream.

- Blood sugar levels are tightly regulated by hormones, primarily insulin and glucagon, to maintain a stable balance.

- High blood sugar levels (hyperglycemia) can occur after eating a meal high in carbohydrates or due to conditions such as diabetes. Prolonged hyperglycemia can damage blood vessels and organs over time.

- Low blood sugar levels (hypoglycemia) can result from skipping meals, excessive exercise, or certain medical conditions. Hypoglycemia can cause symptoms like weakness, dizziness, and confusion.

Insulin:

- Insulin is a hormone produced by the pancreas that helps regulate blood sugar levels by facilitating the uptake of glucose into cells for energy or storage.

- When blood sugar levels rise after eating, the pancreas releases insulin into the bloodstream to signal cells to take up glucose from the blood.

- Insulin also promotes the storage of excess glucose in the liver and muscles as glycogen for later use.

- In addition to regulating blood sugar, insulin plays a role in fat metabolism by promoting the storage of excess calories as fat in adipose tissue.

- Insulin resistance occurs when cells become less responsive to insulin's effects, leading to elevated blood sugar levels and increased insulin production. Insulin resistance is a hallmark of type 2 diabetes and is associated with obesity, metabolic syndrome, and cardiovascular disease.

Relation to Weight Management:

- The balance between blood sugar and insulin is crucial for weight management and overall health.

- Chronically high blood sugar levels and excessive insulin secretion can promote fat storage, particularly around the abdomen.

- Diets high in refined carbohydrates and added sugars can lead to spikes in blood sugar levels and insulin secretion, potentially contributing to weight gain and insulin resistance.

- Low-carbohydrate diets or diets that emphasize whole, unprocessed foods can help stabilize blood sugar levels and improve insulin sensitivity, which may aid in weight loss and metabolic health.

- Regular physical activity, particularly aerobic exercise and resistance training, can help improve insulin sensitivity and regulate blood sugar levels.

Monitoring Blood Sugar and Insulin:

- Monitoring blood sugar levels, particularly for individuals with diabetes or insulin resistance, is essential for managing blood sugar levels and preventing complications.

- Fasting blood sugar, postprandial (after-meal) blood sugar, and hemoglobin A1c (HbA1c) are common tests used to assess blood sugar control over time.

- Insulin levels may also be measured in some cases to assess insulin resistance or insulin production.

- Lifestyle factors such as diet, exercise, stress management, and sleep can all influence blood sugar and insulin levels and should be considered when managing metabolic health.

Maintaining balanced blood sugar and insulin levels through diet, exercise, and lifestyle habits is important for supporting overall health, weight management, and metabolic function.

EMOTIONAL ISSUES RELATED TO OMAD

Following the OMAD (One Meal A Day) diet can present unique emotional challenges for some individuals. While OMAD can offer benefits such as weight loss, improved metabolic health, and simplified meal planning, it may also impact emotional well-being in various ways. Here are some potential emotional issues related to OMAD and strategies for addressing them:

1. Food Obsession and Anxiety:

- **Issue:** Restricting food intake to one meal a day may lead to heightened feelings of food obsession, preoccupation, and anxiety, especially around the timing and content of the single meal.

- **Strategy:** Practice mindfulness and self-awareness to recognize and challenge food-related anxieties. Focus on developing a healthy relationship with food based on balance, moderation, and flexibility. Seek support from a therapist or counselor if food-related anxiety becomes overwhelming.

2. Social Isolation and Disconnection:

- **Issue:** Following OMAD may result in social isolation or feelings of disconnection during social gatherings or meals with family and friends who eat on a different schedule.

- **Strategy:** Communicate openly with loved ones about your dietary choices and preferences. Find ways to participate in social events without compromising your dietary goals, such as focusing on social interaction rather than food or bringing your own OMAD-friendly dish to share. Seek support from like-minded individuals in online communities or local meetups.

3. Emotional Eating Triggers:

- **Issue:** Emotional eating triggers, such as stress, boredom, loneliness, or negative emotions, may become more pronounced when eating patterns are restricted to one meal a day.

- **Strategy:** Develop alternative coping mechanisms for managing emotions, such as practicing mindfulness, engaging in hobbies or activities you enjoy, exercising, journaling, or seeking support from friends or a therapist. Focus on addressing the underlying emotional needs rather than using food as a primary coping mechanism.

4. Mood Swings and Irritability:

- **Issue:** Fluctuations in blood sugar levels and hormonal changes associated with fasting periods may contribute to mood swings, irritability, or emotional instability.

- **Strategy:** Prioritize nutrient-dense foods and balanced meals during your OMAD window to help stabilize blood sugar levels and support mood regulation. Stay hydrated and ensure adequate intake of electrolytes. Consider experimenting with different meal timing or macronutrient ratios to identify patterns that best support your mood and energy levels.

5. Perfectionism and Self-Judgment:

- **Issue:** Striving for perfection or adhering strictly to OMAD guidelines may lead to feelings of guilt, self-judgment, or failure if deviations occur or expectations are not met.

- **Strategy:** Practice self-compassion and flexibility in your approach to OMAD. Allow yourself grace and understanding on days when adherence is challenging or when deviations occur. Focus on progress rather than perfection, and recognize that dietary patterns may vary from day to day based on individual needs and circumstances.

6. Body Image Concerns:

- **Issue:** Following a restrictive eating pattern like OMAD may exacerbate body image concerns or trigger disordered eating behaviors in individuals prone to body dissatisfaction or eating disorders.

- **Strategy:** Prioritize overall health and well-being over appearance or weight-related goals. Focus on nourishing your body with nutrient-dense foods and engaging in activities that promote physical and mental health. Seek support from a healthcare professional, therapist, or support group if body image concerns or disordered eating behaviors arise.

7. Lack of Satisfaction or Enjoyment:

- **Issue:** Consuming all daily calories in a single meal may lead to feelings of deprivation, lack of satisfaction, or reduced enjoyment of food.

- **Strategy:** Focus on making your OMAD meal nutrient-dense, flavorful, and satisfying. Experiment with different foods, flavors, and cooking techniques to enhance enjoyment and satiety. Practice mindful eating by savoring each bite and paying attention to hunger and fullness cues.